GW01111085

THE COMPLETE LONG COVID HANDBOOK

Vol. 1

2nd Edition

Dr. Robert Groysman, MD

info@COVIDinstitute.org

Table of Contents

Medical Disclaimer

The information provided in this book is for educational and informational purposes only and is not intended as medical advice. The content is not a substitute for professional medical expertise or treatment. The contents of this book are not meant to diagnose, treat, or cure any illness. Always seek the advice of your physician or other qualified health providers with any questions you may have regarding a medical condition. Consult your physician if you are pregnant. Never disregard professional medical advice or delay seeking it because of something you have read in this book.

The author and publisher of this book are not responsible for any adverse effects or consequences resulting from the use of any of the suggestions, preparations, or procedures discussed in this book. All readers, especially those taking supplements, prescription, or over-the-counter medications, should consult their physicians before beginning any nutrition, supplement, or lifestyle program. Therefore, no doses have been included in this book.

The information contained herein is provided "*as is*" and without warranties, either express or implied. The authors and publishers disclaim all warranties, express or implied, including, but not limited to, implied warranties of merchantability and fitness for a particular purpose. The author and publisher do not warrant or make any representations regarding the information's use, validity, accuracy, or reliability.

Introduction to the Author

In the evolving landscape of Long COVID treatment, Dr. Robert Groysman, MD, is a pioneering figure who brings clarity and hope to those grappling with this multifaceted condition. As a Diplomate of the American Board of Anesthesiology and the American Board of Pain Medicine, Dr. Groysman combines his extensive credentials with a profound commitment to patient care. He has been treating Long COVID since 2020, even before the term was coined.

Long COVID—also referred to as Long Hauler's or Post-Acute Sequelae of SARS-CoV-2 Infection (PASC)—represents a complex, multisystem condition that can persist Long after the initial COVID-19 infection has resolved. Remarkably, even those who experienced mild or asymptomatic cases of COVID-19 can develop Long COVID, which often presents with chronic fatigue, brain fog, taste and smell abnormalities, neuropathies, abdominal pain, bloating, chest pain, and vibration sensations.

In this groundbreaking book, Dr. Groysman shares his deep expertise and innovative approaches to treating Long COVID. His journey into this field began with applying stellate ganglion block (SGB) techniques to address the common dysautonomia witnessed in Long COVID patients. Recognizing the need for a comprehensive approach, he has expanded his treatments to include stellate ganglion procedure, EAT therapy, external vagus nerve stimulation, nicotine patches (14 days or less), prescription medications, supplements, herbals, and IV therapy.

Dr. Groysman's practice sets the pace and evolves the treatment modalities used to treat Long COVID. His dedication to repurposing existing medications and supplements underscores his commitment to tackling the systemic and chronic nature of Long COVID, which involves dysautonomia, mitochondrial dysfunction, excess histamine, and gut dysbiosis. Researchers estimate that over 200 symptoms can occur in Long COVID. These symptoms could persist for months or years, affecting multiple organs, and recovery can be prolonged; Dr. Groysman's comprehensive approach offers invaluable insights and hope.

In this book, Dr. Groysman outlines his methodologies and successes and provides a beacon of hope for those suffering from Long COVID. His innovative and organized strategies and compassionate care demonstrate that while Long COVID poses significant challenges, there is a path forward, marked by determination, expertise, and the relentless pursuit of better treatments. Dr. Groysman's work is a testament to the power of advanced medical care and the unwavering hope that we can overcome the challenges of Long COVID.

What is New in this 2nd Edition?

Dr. Groysman has done it again! Just when it seemed that ***The Complete Long COVID Handbook, Volume 1*** covered everything, new information emerged. Long COVID is a constantly evolving condition, and that's exactly what this second edition addresses—keeping you up-to-date with the latest developments.

New Chapters and Sections Added

a. Brain fog section added

b. Neuropathies section added including small fiber neuropathies (SFN)

c. Gastroparesis section added

d. Tinnitus section added

2. Autoimmunity section greatly expanded.
3. New lotting **chapter** added including a section on microclots.
4. Oxidation and reduction rewritten to make it easier to understand.
5. All images are bigger and flipped on side when needed to make them easier to read.
6. New intermittent fasting **chapter** added.
7. New chronic fatigue (ME/CFS) **chapter** added.
8. EAT questionnaire added.
9. Added a new **chapter** on Vitamin D, phosphorus, and calcium added.
10. Accelerated aging, why, and how to treat **chapter.**

11. EDS **chapter** expanded.
12. New Ebstein Barr Virus (EBV) **chapter** added.
13. Pediatric symptoms chapter expanded.
14. Histamine **chapter** greatly expanded including methylation's role in the **metabolism of histamine.**
15. Expanded nicotine patch section.
16. Every chapter has extra references added.

And a few more surprises...

Foreword

Long COVID has emerged as one of the most complex and challenging medical conditions of our time. Over the past few years, it has confounded patients and healthcare providers alike, presenting a wide array of symptoms that vary from mild to debilitating. Understanding this condition is crucial, not only for those who suffer from it but also for the medical professionals striving to offer effective care.

This book, the first in a comprehensive series examining the causes and treatments of Long COVID. Designed for both patients and doctors, this book offers an in-depth exploration of Long COVID, breaking down the condition into understandable segments. You will gain knowledge of the risk factors, the underlying causes, and the various treatment options available. Importantly, this book is not just about theory; it's about practical, actionable strategies that can be implemented in real-life scenarios.

As you embark on this journey through the pages of this book, you will discover not only the science behind Long COVID but also the personal insights that come from years of hands-on experience. My goal is to help you understand what is happening inside your body, why you feel the way you do, and to validate that your symptoms are real and not merely "in your head." Long COVID is a genuine medical condition, and this book aims to shed light on its many facets.

While treatment options are discussed in detail, I have deliberately refrained from prescribing specific dosages or one-size-fits-all solutions. Treatment is highly individual, and what works for one person may not work for another. This book is meant to serve as a guide, offering a clear strategy that you can discuss with your healthcare provider to tailor the best approach for your unique situation. Natural treatments, though often beneficial, can be harmful if not used correctly, and it is essential to make informed decisions in collaboration with your provider.

Through the experience of treating Long COVID and related conditions for over four years, I have seen the positive impact of a well-structured, personalized treatment plan. This book is designed to help you focus and organize your treatment into a working plan that you can share with your healthcare provider. While all the information presented is evidence-based, it is also enriched by my personal experiences and the lessons I have learned in the field.

This book is more than just a guide; it is a tool to empower you in your journey towards better health. Whether you are a patient seeking relief or a doctor looking to expand your knowledge, this book provides the wisdom and resources needed to understand and effectively treat Long COVID.

The goal of this book is to focus and organize your treatments better. Most people hunt and peck from social media groups and google for treatments. This would be similar to trying to construct a jig saw puzzle, but using several different puzzles for the pieces at the same time. What kind of final result will you get? It just doesn't work.

Long COVID is similar to describing a multi-car pileup. In each vehicle, people will have diverse injuries. One will have a broken arm. Another patient will have a bruised chest. Another will have burns on the leg. Despite a common cause, each person's treatment plan will be unique.

Please take a look at the other books in this series, including:

- **Volume 2**: The Complete Long COVID Handbook: Dysautonomia
- **Volume 3**: The Complete Long COVID Handbook: Mitochondrial Dysfunction
- **Volume 4**: The Complete Long COVID Handbook: Gut Dysbiosis
- **Volume 5**: The Complete Long COVID Handbook: Histamine and Mast Cell Activation

Introduction to Long Covid

Long COVID, also referred to as *Post-Acute Sequelae of SARS-CoV-2* (PASC) infection, Long Hauler's condition, as well as many other names. It is a condition characterized by either the persistence or the development of new symptoms following the acute phase of a COVID-19 infection. You must have recovered from COVID-19 before you can have Long COVID. There is no agreement on defining what this syndrome/illness/disease should be called or how to describe it. One definition focuses on the symptoms, while another centers around its timing.

These symptoms can last for several weeks, months, or years, significantly impacting your quality of life. Long COVID includes a broad range of symptoms that can affect multiple organ systems, including respiratory, cardiovascular, neurological, and gastrointestinal systems. This book will review possible causes, mechanisms, testing, and treatment strategies.

Because Long COVID has over 200 symptoms and the presentation of symptoms is variable, I primarily focus on four causes and how much each cause contributes to the symptoms of Long COVID. It is not productive to chase symptoms of Long COVID. Chasing symptoms is acceptable in the short term while treating the causes, but I often find it similar to a game of *Whack-a-Mole*. You knock one symptom down, and another one pops up.

Most treatments provided out there for Long COVID are symptom-driven and generally apply to any chronic illness, such as not pushing yourself, getting mental health therapy, *etc*. Despite some of the treatments that I use being experimental, they are evidence-based and are backed by studies and my personal experiences. I focus on the causes first. I see this as a unique way to treat Long COVID. I assign the symptoms to each cause responsible for Long COVID. Each cause contributes a unique percentage to each patient. Consequently, it creates a kind of profile or fingerprint for each patient. No two treatments are alike. It would be similar to coming up to a 5-car pileup accident. Everyone was involved in a car accident, but everyone has different problems. One has a leg fracture. Another has a bruise on her forehead. Yet another's chest hurts. A fourth has a bleeding arm. The last one has abdominal pain. Even though everyone has had the same car accident, the approach, testing, and treatment for each will differ. In a similar fashion, I approach the treatment of Long COVID.

By treating the causes, we can resolve each cause's contribution to Long COVID. I view the other potential causes as consequences rather than the causes such as autoimmune conditions. While I have seen phenotypes created based on the symptom analysis for Long COVID, they often do not agree from study to study. Instead, I prefer to examine the causes and what contributes to each person's symptoms. My system works. I have treated many patients using this system, which has proven successful for the last few years. It is organized and doesn't rely on fads, hunting and pecking solutions, or looking for the next best thing to try. You also will not find any pseudoscience treatments in this book.

Specifically, I examine causes such as:

1. **Dysautonomia**
2. **Mitochondrial dysfunction**
3. **Gut dysbiosis**
4. **Mast cell dysfunction**

Don't worry if you are unaware of these medical terms. I will explain how each can cause Long COVID and how you can improve from each one. There are other theories on other causes, but I will discuss how I treat Long COVID, the related conditions using these four, and how all the different causes are actually consequences of these four causes.

Long Covid Risk Factors

Long COVID comprises many symptoms that can vary significantly between individuals. These symptoms vary because each person with Long COVID contributes differently from the four causes. Autoimmune conditions and blood clots are consequences of the four causes rather than the causes themselves.

Risk Factors for Getting Long COVID

Understanding who is most at risk for developing Long COVID is vital for prevention and treatment. Having one of these risk factors does not guarantee you will come down with Long COVID. This section reviews the current epidemiological data, including prevalence rates, demographic factors, and potential risk factors such as preexisting health conditions, severity of initial infection, and sociodemographic variables. All of these can potentially increase your risk of getting Long COVID, but it is not a guarantee that you will get it. Primarily, any condition that is associated with dysautonomia or autonomic neuropathy increases your risk. The bottom line is that having preexisting autonomic nervous system damage or defect is a significant risk factor for Long COVID. A risk factor is a risk, not a guarantee that you will get Long COVID. The risk for Long COVID remains even after you recover.

Risk factors are associated with preexisting damage to the autonomic nervous system, also known as autonomic neuropathy or dysautonomia. The conditions causing this situation are listed below:

- Preexisting herpes family viral infections such as *Cytomegalovirus* (CMV), *Ebstein-Barr Virus* (EBV), *Human Herpes Virus* (HHV-6, roseola infantum), HHV-7 (roseola infantum, exanthem subitem (ES), or 6th disease), chicken pox (varicella herpes zoster)

- Prior Lyme disease or other spirochete infections
- *Erlos-Danlos Syndrome* (EDS)
- Preexisting autoimmunity such as *Crohn's* disease, ulcerative colitis, rheumatoid arthritis, lupus/SLE, Sjogren's syndrome
- Preexisting *Dysautonomia – Postural Orthostatic Tachycardia Syndrome* (POTS), Myalgic encephalomyelitis/chronic fatigue syndrome (ME/CFS), Post Traumatic Stress Disorder (PTSD), diabetes mellitus
- Vitamin B6 toxicity

In addition, there are some risk factors for other reasons:

- Female >> male gender
- Age being under 50 years old
- Number of COVID-19 infections (risk for Long COVID increases by 5% each time)
- Preexisting gut dysbiosis
- Having five or more symptoms during the 1st week of an acute COVID-19 infection
- Physical or emotional stress and traumatic events

References:

1. Subramanian, A., Nirantharakumar, K., Hughes, S. *et al.* Symptoms and risk factors for Long COVID in non-hospitalized adults. *Nat Med* **28**, 1706–1714 (2022). https://DOI.org/10.1038/s41591-022-01909-w

2. Asadi-Pooya AA, Akbari A, Emami A, Lotfi M, Rostamihosseinkhani M, Nemati H, Barzegar Z, Kabiri M, Zeraatpisheh Z, Farjoud-Kouhanjani M, Jafari A, Sasannia F, Ashrafi S, Nazeri M, Nasiri S, Shahisavandi M. Risk Factors Associated with Long COVID Syndrome: A Retrospective Study. Iran J Med Sci. 2021 Nov;46(6):428-436. DOI: 10.30476/ijms.2021.92080.2326. PMID: 34840383; PMCID: PMC8611223.

3. Munipalli B, Ma Y, Li Z, et al. Risk factors for post-acute sequelae of COVID-19: Survey results from a tertiary care hospital. Journal of Investigative Medicine. 2023;71(8):896-906. DOI:10.1177/10815589231190560

4. Jeffrey, K., Woolford, L., Maini, R., Basetti, S., Batchelor, A., Weatherill, D., et al. (2024). Prevalence and risk factors for Long COVID among adults in Scotland using electronic health records: A national, retrospective, observational cohort study. EClinicalMedicine.

   https://DOI.org/10.1016/j.eclinm.2024.102590

5. Müller, S. A., Isaaka, L., Mumm, R., Scheidt-Nave, C., Heldt, K., Schuster, A., et al. (2023). Prevalence and risk factors for Long COVID and post-COVID-19 condition in Africa: A systematic review. The Lancet Global Health.

   https://DOI.org/10.1016/S2214-109X(23)00384-4

6. Batiha, G.ES., Al-kuraishy, H.M., Al-Gareeb, A.I. *et al.* Pathophysiology of Post-COVID syndromes: a new perspective. *Virol J* **19**, 158 (2022).

   https://DOI.org/10.1186/s12985-022-01891-2

7. Davis, H.E., McCorkell, L., Vogel, J.M. *et al.* Long COVID: major findings, mechanisms, and recommendations. *Nat Rev Microbiol* **21**, 133–146 (2023).

https://DOI.org/10.1038/s41579-022-00846-2

Causes of Long Covid

The risks listed above do not cause Long COVID. While the exact mechanisms underlying Long COVID are not entirely understood, several theories have been proposed. This section explores these theories, supported by current research findings, to provide an all-inclusive understanding of the potential biological underpinnings of Long COVID. I will concentrate on the four marked with a * because I believe these to be the primary four causes, with everything else as secondary or contributing.

Multiple Theories of Causes

- * Dysautonomia/vagus nerve dysfunction
- * Mitochondrial dysfunction
- * Excess histamine/mast cell degranulation
- * Gut dysbiosis
- Autoimmunity/immune dysregulation
- Thrombosis/Blood clotting
    - While I am aware of the microclots theory, because the treatment involves using clopidogrel (antiplatelet), aspirin, and apixaban (anticoagulant), which significantly increases your risk for bleeding, I have not incorporated this theory into my practice. Another reason is that the testing for microclots is not conclusive.
- Chronic inflammation

- Viral persistence – there is evidence that COVID-19 can persist in some people for up to 14 months.
    - Viral remnants – viral protein persistence
- Reactivation of latent viruses or infections (Herpes simplex, CMV, EBV, Parvovirus B19, Lyme, HHV-6A/B, varicella zoster - chicken pox)

Of course, stress and anxiety would not cause Long COVID, but it can make symptoms worse or cause flares of your symptoms.

My diagnostic and treatment protocols are not just practical and make a difference. They've brought significant improvements in health and function to many who suffer from Long COVID and COVID vaccine injuries, also known as Long vax. I hope this book will help you as much as I relished writing it.

Why focus on just these four causes? When determining a cause, I assess the reliability and validity of a test or diagnosis and then consider the risks associated with the treatment. If a test or diagnosis lacks validity or reliability or the treatment poses too significant a risk, I won't use it. "First, do no harm." This principle is at the core of my practice. I take it seriously and wholeheartedly believe in it.

Each cause can elaborate on many symptoms and consequences of Long COVID, addressing downstream issues such as autoimmune disorders, immune system dysfunction, chronic inflammation, leaky gut syndrome, malabsorption, and vagus nerve dysfunction.

Why not viral persistence? Viral remnants can remain persistent after recovery from acute COVID infection. These remnants, including spike proteins, are fundamental but reside inside cells. Rather than attempting the impossible task of eliminating these remnants, I focus on improving cellular health through processes like autophagy and mitophagy in damaged cells and mitochondria.

Why not microclots? While clots can occur during COVID and Long COVID, the clinical significance of microclots is not transparent yet. The clots I am concerned about—*e.g.,* deep vein thrombosis, pulmonary embolus, heart attacks, and strokes—have serious consequences. Moreover, microclots also occur in other chronic illnesses like diabetes mellitus Type 2, Alzheimer's, Parkinson's, and rheumatoid arthritis, yet patients are not routinely placed on anticoagulants or antiplatelet medications unless they're at significant risk for major clots. Triple therapy poses a severe risk of bleeding. Medications like apixaban and clopidogrel can inhibit clotting and platelets, but I believe the risk of uncontrolled bleeding outweighs the uncertain benefits of preventing microclots. Above all else, first, do no harm—this is an integral part of the *Hippocratic Oath.*

Why not autoimmune or apheresis? I do consider autoimmune conditions, including autoantibodies. Doing HELP apheresis doesn't solve the cause of these antibodies, and the treatments would need to be done for the rest of your life. Apheresis can be risky because blood is removed, anticoagulated, and then reinfused. Many possible complications can occur because of this, including infections, bleeding, and clots.

Why not reactivated Ebstein Barr Virus, Lyme disease (Borrelia), Babesia, or Bartonella? While these can contribute to the symptoms of Long COVID, I do not believe these are a cause of Long COVID. These conditions have been found in the past in immunocompromised people, yet the presentation is significantly different from Long COVID. The symptoms of reacted EBV can mimic some symptoms of Long Covid, but it is treated differently from Long Covid. I will address this in a later chapter. Lyme disease can remain untreated, because you didn't know you had it, or be a chronic infection. Again, this is not Long Covid, and would need to be treated as Lyme disease.

References:

- Su Y, Yuan D, Chen DG, Davis MM, Goldman JD, Heath JR. Multiple early factors anticipate post-acute COVID-19 sequelae. *Cell.* 2022;184(2):265-283.e18. DOI:10.1016/j.cell.2022.01.014.

- Davis, H.E., McCorkell, L., Vogel, J.M. *et al.* Long COVID: Major findings, mechanisms, and recommendations. *Nat Rev Microbiol* **21**, 133–146 (2023). https://DOI.org/10.1038/s41579-022-00846-2

Questionnaire to Fill Out Before You Go to Your Doctor

1. Have you been infected with COVID-19 virus: list dates;

   ____

2. Have you been vaccinated against COVID-19? List dates and manufacturer if known (M=Moderna, P = Pfizer, J = Johnson & Johnson)

   ____

3. Do you have PoTS? MCAS? Chronic fatigue (ME/CFS)?

4. Risk factors: Have you had Lyme disease? EBV (mono)? Crohn/s disease, ulcerative colitis, celiac disease.

5. What symptoms do you currently have? <u>(Circle all that apply)</u>

   a. **Systemic (entire body):** fatigue, post-exertional malaise, weakness, temperature dysregulation

   b. **Neurological**: brain fog, concentration issues, loss of taste/smell, abnormal taste/smell, memory problems, insomnia, pins and needles, vibrations, neuropathies, dizziness, numbness, headaches, tinnitus, seizures, tremors

   c. **Psychiatric**: anxiety, irritability, depression, PTSD, tearfulness

   d. **Cardiovascular** (heart/blood): tachycardia, palpitations, chest pain, inflamed blood vessels

e. **Pulmonary** (lungs): shortness of breath, dry cough, breathing difficulty

f. **Ear, nose, eyes, and throat:** sore throat, blurry vision/change in vision, lump in throat/hoarseness, sensitivity to light or sound

g. **Gastrointestinal**: abdominal cramps, bloating, diarrhea, nausea/vomiting, GERD

h. **Dermatologic** (skin): rashes, petechiae, itchy skin

i. **Musculoskeletal**: chest tightness, muscle aches, joint pains, muscle spasms

j. **Reproductive**: period changes, heavy periods, sexual dysfunction, bladder control issues, testicular pain.

k. **Immunologic**: increased allergies, new allergies, shingles, EBV reactivation

6. What blood work have you had? (circle)

a. CBC with differential, basic metabolic panel, liver function tests, D-dimer, CRP, TSH, Free T3, Homocysteine level, HbA1C, Troponin, pro-BNP, vitamin D, vitamin B12, ferritin, 24hr urine N-methylhistamine, ANA, lupus anticoagulant.

7. What over-the-counter supplements have you tried? (do not list anything not on the list)

a. Resveratrol, quercetin, co Q-10, omega 3 fatty acids, magnesium, vitamin D, vitamin B12/B complex, NAC, melatonin, probiotics, nattokinase/serropeptase/lumbrokinase, bromelain, L-arginine, L-citrulline, vitamin C, nigella sativa (black seed oil), PEA/luteolin, curcumin, lactoferrin, selenium, zinc, iron.

8. What prescription medications have you tried?

a. Guanfacine, Mestinon (pyridostigmine), Low-Dose Naltrexone (LDN), ivermectin, hydroxychloroquine, colchicine, Cetirizine (Zyrtec), famotidine/Pepcid, nadolol, midodrine, antidepressants, benzodiazepines, Maraviroc, Paxlovid, triple anticoagulant therapy (Clopidogrel 75mg + Aspirin 75mg) once a day, and a direct oral anticoagulant (Apixaban) 5mg twice a day. pantoprazole 40 mg/day for gastric protection.

Other:_______________________________________

9. Do you use a vagus nerve stimulator?
10. Have you tried the nicotine patch?
11. Have you had an SGB (stellate ganglion block)?
    a. Was it 1 level or 2 (one-shot or 2 on the same side)?
    b. Was it done with an ultrasound?
    c. Did you have *Horner's* syndrome (red eye, small pupil, droopy eye, stuffy nostril)?
12. What other treatments have you tried?

COVID-19 VACCINE INJURIES

COVID-19 vaccine injuries refer to adverse events after receiving a COVID-19 vaccine. While COVID-19 vaccines have been thought to be safe for the vast majority of people, some individuals may experience adverse reactions. I surmise that the spike protein causes the mechanism behind these injuries, whether injected directly into the muscle or manufactured from the mRNA of your own cells. Damage comes from the spike protein, is inside the cell cytoplasm and interacts with mitochondria. The SARS-COV-2 viral proteins can damage mitochondria's own DNA (mtDNA), cause extensive oxidative stress damage, and produce abnormal proteins that interfere with mitochondrial function. The damage that remains in Long Covid is not as widespread as from the actual COVID infection. I do not believe that this effect is permanent.

It is essential for you to know that I am neither for nor against COVID vaccines. I provide information based on the available evidence and my experiences. These reactions are natural and have affected thousands; no one should feel dismissed or gaslighted when visiting their physicians. So, if you haven't heard this said yet by a physician/doctor, I believe you and your symptoms are real and not in your head. You can review more complications from here:

https://COVIDinstitute.org/COVID-vaccine-injuries/

Outside of common side effects and allergy to the vaccine, there have been several reported complications in the literature. I understand that these complications directly result from damage to mitochondria. Damaging mitochondria in nerves can cause neuropathies, neuritis, and dysautonomia.

Myocarditis and Pericarditis

Inflammation of the heart muscle (myocarditis) or the lining around the heart (pericarditis) has been reported, primarily in younger males following mRNA vaccines. These cases are generally rare and often resolved with treatment.

Thrombosis with Thrombocytopenia Syndrome (TTS) / Blood Clots

A rare but severe condition involving blood clots with low platelet counts. This condition requires immediate medical attention. It is not associated with microclots.

Guillain-Barré Syndrome (GBS)

It is a rare condition where the immune system attacks the nerves, potentially causing muscle weakness and paralysis. It has been associated with the *Johnson & Johnson* vaccine but remains extremely rare.

Bell's Palsy

It is temporary facial paralysis or weakness on one side of the face. Cases have been reported but are rare and typically resolve on their own.

Immune Thrombocytopenia (ITP)

ITP is a rare condition characterized by a low platelet count, which can lead to bruising and bleeding.

Chronic Conditions

There are reports of chronic symptoms or conditions developing after vaccination, but these are still being studied for potential causality and prevalence. These can present similar to Long COVID.

Reporting claims

Over 270 million Americans were vaccinated for COVID. Among them, up to 13,000 injury claims have been filed so far. According to the Informed

Consent Action Network (ICAN), 7.7% of the v-safe users, a website run by the CDC, use a vaccine safety monitoring system. Approximately 800,000 people have reported seeking medical attention via telehealth appointments, urgent care clinics, emergency room interventions, or hospitalizations following the COVID-19 vaccine. The *Centers for Disease Control* (CDC) and the *Federal Drug Administration* (FDA) also maintain a *Vaccine Adverse Event Reporting System* (VAERS).

If you suspect you have been injured after receiving a COVID vaccine, you can submit a claim to the National Vaccine Injury Compensation Program here:

https://www.hrsa.gov/vaccine-compensation

References:

1. https://fingfx.thomsonreuters.com/gfx/legaldocs/dwvkaljdkvm/CICP COMPLAINT.pdf

2. https://www.cdc.gov/vaccinesafety/ensuringsafety/monitoring/v-safe/index.html

3. Bluemke, D. A. (2023). COVID-19 vaccines and myocardial injury. Radiology. https://DOI.org/10.1148/radiol.232244

4. National Academies of Sciences, Engineering, and Medicine. (2024). Evidence Review of the Adverse Effects of COVID-19 Vaccination and Intramuscular Vaccine Administration. Washington, DC: The National Academies Press. https://DOI.org/10.17226/27746

5. An QJ, Qin DA, Pei JX. Reactive arthritis after COVID-19 vaccination. Hum Vaccin Immunother. 2021 Sep 2;17(9):2954-2956. DOI: 10.1080/21645515.2021.1920274. Epub 2021 May 25. PMID: 34033732; PMCID: PMC8381833.

6. Gómez de Terreros Caro G, Gil Díaz S, Pérez Alé M, Martínez Gimeno ML. Bell's palsy following COVID-19 vaccination: a case report. Neurologia (Engl Ed). 2021 Sep;36(7):567-568. DOI:

10.1016/j.nrleng.2021.04.002. Epub 2021 Jul 22. PMID: 34330676; PMCID: PMC8295024.

7. Martin-Villares C, Vazquez-Feito A, Gonzalez-Gimeno MJ, de la Nogal-Fernandez B. Bell's palsy following a single dose of mRNA SARS-CoV-2 vaccine: a case report. J Neurol. 2022 Jan;269(1):47-48. DOI: 10.1007/s00415-021-10617-3. Epub 2021 May 25. PMID: 34032902; PMCID: PMC8143982.

8. Rao SJ, Khurana S, Murthy G, Dawson ET, Jazebi N, Haas CJ. A case of Guillain-Barre syndrome following Pfizer COVID-19 vaccine. J Community Hosp Intern Med Perspect. 2021 Sep 20;11(5):597-600. DOI:

   10.1080/20009666.2021.1954284. PMID: 34567447;

   PMCID: PMC8462911.

9. Finsterer J, Scorza FA, Scorza CA. Post SARS-CoV-2 vaccination Guillain-Barre syndrome in 19 patients. Clinics (Sao Paulo). 2021 Oct 11;76:e3286. DOI:

   10.6061/clinics/2021/e3286. PMID: 34644738; PMCID: PMC8478139.

10. Patone, M., Mei, X. W., Handunnetthi, L., Dixon, S., Zaccardi, F., Shankar-Hari, M., Watkinson, P., Khunti, K., Harnden, A., Coupland, C. A. C., & Hippisley-Cox, J. (2021). Risks of myocarditis, pericarditis, and cardiac arrhythmias associated with COVID-19 vaccination or SARS-CoV-2 infection. *Circulation*. https://DOI.org/10.1161/CIRCULATIONAHA.121.056135

11. Kim IC, Kim H, Lee HJ, Kim JY, Kim JY. Cardiac Imaging of Acute Myocarditis Following COVID-19 mRNA Vaccination. J Korean Med Sci. 2021 Aug 16;36(32):e229. DOI: 10.3346/jkms.2021.36.e229. PMID: 34402228; PMCID: PMC8369314.

Can Long COVID be Prevented?

It depends on who you ask. Ask the CDC or Google search; without hesitation, the answer is COVID vaccination is the best available tool to prevent Long COVID. Additionally, getting vaccinated after recovering from Long COVID, again vaccination is mentioned in order to avoid Long COVID. Take that as you will.

According to one study, metformin, especially if taken early during COVID infection, can help reduce the occurrence of Long COVID.

Another study points to antihistamines, including both H1 and H2 blockers. H1 blockers are significant. Finally, Paxlovid has been suggested as a means to reduce the risk of Long COVID.

One study suggested Serotonin Reuptake Inhibitors (SSRIs) can also help minimize the risk of Long COVID.

- Some masks have been shown to be helpful like N95 or KN95.
- Medical grade HEPA filters can also be helpful.
- According to one study, **metformin**, a medicine prescribed for diabetes to control blood sugar, can help. If taken early during COVID infection, it can help reduce the Long COVID.
- Another study points to antihistamines (H1) blockers like Benadryl® or Zyrtec® can help reduce long COVID.
- Paxlovid, a medicine that kills viruses, has been suggested as a means to reduce the risk of Long COVID.

- One study suggested Serotonin Reuptake Inhibitors (SSRIs) can also help minimize the risk of Long COVID.
- I **will not** talk about Ivermectin in this book because I have not found it to be relevant in treating Long COVID.
- Some nasal sprays have been shown to help by being a barrier.

Nasal Sprays used for Covid Prevention

1. Taffix (Low pH Hypromellose)

- **Mechanism**: Taffix creates a mechanical barrier in the nasal cavity. The spray forms a gel-like layer, lowering the pH and blocking viral particles from attaching to nasal cells. The low pH environment helps inactivate viruses, including SARS-CoV-2.
- **Theoretical Efficacy**: By reducing viral load and making the environment inhospitable to the virus, Taffix could theoretically lower the chances of infection.
- **Real-life Efficacy**: Clinical studies suggest Taffix can reduce the risk of COVID-19 by up to 78% in high-risk environments. A study noted that participants who used the spray regularly had fewer infections compared to the control group.
- https://pubmed.ncbi.nlm.nih.gov/33759682/

2. Enovid/VirX/Fabrispray (Nitric Oxide Nasal Spray - NONS)

- **Mechanism**: Nitric oxide has antiviral properties and acts by disrupting viral replication and neutralizing viral particles upon contact. NONS works by releasing nitric oxide, which can kill SARS-CoV-2 in the nasal cavity.
- **Theoretical Efficacy**: NONS could reduce the viral load in the upper respiratory tract, theoretically reducing transmission and severity of infection.

- **Real-life Efficacy**: Early studies showed that it could reduce viral load by 95% within 24 hours and completely clear the virus in some patients within 72 hours. It has been found to lower infection rates when used prophylactically in high-risk settings.
- https://www.ncbi.nlm.nih.gov/pmc/articles/PMC8117664/

3. Xlear Nasal Spray (Xylitol and Grapefruit Seed Extract)

- **Mechanism**: Xlear uses xylitol, a sugar alcohol, and grapefruit seed extract, which can block viral adhesion to nasal membranes. Xylitol also promotes moisture and maintains a protective barrier in the nasal passages.
- **Theoretical Efficacy**: Xylitol has shown promise in inhibiting bacterial growth, and this effect could theoretically extend to preventing viral infections like COVID-19.
- **Real-life Efficacy**: A clinical trial (NCT04858620) is investigating its effectiveness in reducing COVID-19 viral load. Preliminary evidence suggests that regular use of Xlear may reduce the risk of viral infections, though more robust data are needed.
- https://clinicaltrials.gov/study/NCT04858620
- https://www.ncbi.nlm.nih.gov/pmc/articles/PMC7645297/

4. Bentolite Clay Nasal Spray

- **Mechanism**: Bentolite clay may trap viral particles, preventing them from entering cells by forming a physical barrier in the nasal mucosa.
- **Theoretical Efficacy**: The physical entrapment of viral particles could theoretically reduce the chances of SARS-CoV-2 entering the nasal cells, preventing infection.

- **Real-life Efficacy**: While it's a promising idea, there is limited clinical data on the effectiveness of Bentolite clay in real-world settings for COVID-19. Studies are still ongoing.
- https://www.news-medical.net/news/20210719/Inhibition-of-SARS-CoV-2-by-bentonite-based-nasal-spray.aspx

5. Iota-Carrageenan Nasal Spray

- **Mechanism**: Carrageenan is a natural compound derived from red seaweed, which forms a gel-like barrier in the nasal cavity, trapping viruses and preventing their attachment to mucosal cells.
- **Theoretical Efficacy**: By trapping viral particles, iota-carrageenan could theoretically reduce infection risk by preventing viral entry into cells.
- **Real-life Efficacy**: Clinical studies suggest it reduces the viral load and severity of COVID-19. In one study, individuals using iota-carrageenan nasal spray had a lower incidence of SARS-CoV-2 infections compared to a control group.
- https://www.ncbi.nlm.nih.gov/pmc/articles/PMC8493111/

6. Hydrogen Peroxide Nasal Spray

- **Mechanism**: Hydrogen peroxide has antiseptic properties that could theoretically neutralize viral particles by oxidative damage.
- **Theoretical Efficacy**: The virus-killing effect of hydrogen peroxide could reduce viral load in the nasal cavity, helping to prevent infection.
- **Real-life Efficacy**: Limited real-life data suggest potential benefits, but there is caution regarding safety and long-term use, as it can cause nasal irritation and mucosal damage if used excessively.

- https://www.e-epih.org/upload/pdf/epih-43-e2021032.pdf

7. Povidone-Iodine Nasal Spray

- **Mechanism**: Povidone-iodine is a broad-spectrum antiseptic. It kills viruses by disrupting their outer structure, preventing them from infecting cells.

- **Theoretical Efficacy**: Povidone-iodine has shown high effectiveness in killing coronaviruses, making it a promising agent for COVID-19 prevention.

- **Real-life Efficacy**: Studies demonstrate that povidone-iodine nasal sprays can reduce the viral load significantly when used pre- or post-exposure. It is recommended in some protocols as part of a prophylactic regimen for healthcare workers.

- https://pubmed.ncbi.nlm.nih.gov/34724213/

8. Covixyl (Ethyl Lauroyl Arginine Hydrochloride - ELAH)

- **Mechanism**: Covixyl forms a protective film in the nasal cavity, blocking viruses from adhering to mucosal cells. The compound creates a barrier that prevents SARS-CoV-2 from binding to ACE2 receptors.

- **Theoretical Efficacy**: Covixyl's ability to block viral entry makes it theoretically effective in reducing the risk of infection when applied before exposure.

- **Real-life Efficacy**: Early studies show that Covixyl can reduce infection rates in high-risk environments, but large-scale clinical trials are still pending.

- https://www.ncbi.nlm.nih.gov/pmc/articles/PMC9313533/

9. Carragelose Nasal Spray (Marinomed Biotech AG)

- **Mechanism**: Carragelose (iota-carrageenan) is derived from red algae and forms a protective gel barrier in the nasal cavity. It works by trapping viral particles, including SARS-CoV-2, which prevents the virus from attaching to host cells and initiating infection.

- **Theoretical Efficacy**: The gel barrier traps viruses in the nasal passages, effectively reducing viral load. Carragelose has been shown to neutralize various respiratory viruses, including coronaviruses, making it theoretically effective against COVID-19.

- **Real-life Efficacy**: Clinical trials indicate that Carragelose nasal spray can reduce the incidence of COVID-19 in high-risk populations. It has been found to reduce viral loads in infected individuals and prevent the onset of symptoms in pre-symptomatic cases. One study showed that Carragelose users had a significantly lower infection rate compared to a control group during high-exposure periods.

- https://www.ncbi.nlm.nih.gov/pmc/articles/PMC8493111/

10. VirX™ (Altimmune)

- **Mechanism**: VirX™ is a nasal vaccine developed by Altimmune. It delivers a dose of a vaccine into the nasal mucosa, stimulating both local and systemic immune responses. This includes the activation of mucosal immunity, which is crucial in blocking respiratory pathogens like SARS-CoV-2 at the entry point.

- **Theoretical Efficacy**: By stimulating the mucosal immune system directly, VirX™ could prevent SARS-CoV-2 from establishing an infection in the respiratory tract. The vaccine formulation could also trigger robust systemic immunity, providing long-lasting protection against COVID-19.

- **Real-life Efficacy**: Preclinical studies demonstrated that VirX™ induces strong mucosal and systemic immune responses against

SARS-CoV-2. However, as of the latest updates, human clinical trials were still ongoing. Early results from animal studies show that the nasal vaccine could prevent infection and transmission of COVID-19 effectively, but more clinical data are needed to confirm this in humans.

- https://ir.altimmune.com/news-releases/news-release-details/adcovidtm-altimmunes-single-dose-intranasal-covid-19-vaccine

Each of these nasal sprays operates by different mechanisms, from physically blocking the virus to chemically neutralizing it. While their theoretical efficacy is promising, more clinical trials and real-world data are needed to fully establish their effectiveness in preventing COVID-19.

References:

1. Bramante, C. T., Buse, J. B., Liebovitz, D. M., Nicklas, J. M., Puskarich, M. A., Cohen, K., et al. (2023). Outpatient treatment of COVID-19 and incidence of post-COVID-19 condition over 10 months (COVID-OUT): A multicentre, randomized, quadruple-blind, parallel-group, phase 3 trial. *The Lancet Infectious Diseases*. Published June 08, 2023. https://DOI.org/10.1016/S1473-3099(23)00299-2

2. Mashauri HL. COVID-19 Histamine theory: Why antihistamines should be incorporated as the basic component in COVID-19 management? Health Sci Rep. 2023 Feb 7;6(2):e1109. DOI: 10.1002/hsr2.1109. PMID: 36778771; PMCID: PMC9903129.

3. Xie Y, Choi T, Al-Aly Z. Association of Treatment with Nirmatrelvir and the Risk of Post-COVID-19 Condition. JAMA Intern Med. 2023 Jun 1;183(6):554-564. DOI: 10.1001/jamainternmed.2023.0743. PMID: 36951829; PMCID: PMC10037200.

4. Sidky H, Sahner DK, Girvin AT, Hotaling N, Michael SG, Gersing K. Assessing the Effect of Selective Serotonin Reuptake Inhibitors in the Prevention of Post-Acute Sequelae of COVID-19. medRxiv [Preprint]. 2023 Feb 10:2022.11.09.22282142. DOI:

10.1101/2022.11.09.22282142. Update in: Comput Struct Biotechnol J. 2024 Jan 09;24:115-125. DOI: 10.1016/j.csbj.2023.12.045. PMID: 36380766; PMCID: PMC9665345.

5. Narayan Y, Chatterjee S, Agrawal A, Bhardwaj R. Effectiveness of N95 Mask in Preventing COVID-19 Transmission. Trans Indian Natl Acad Eng. 2023;8(2):253-262. doi: 10.1007/s41403-023-00394-y. Epub 2023 Feb 23. PMID: 36851950; PMCID: PMC9947910.

Long COVID Symptoms

Because Long COVID has over 200 possible symptoms, determining if you are feeling sick, mainly from Long COVID, is imperative. Common medical conditions still occur despite Long COVID. This section describes the criteria used to diagnose Long COVID. It is essential to note that Long COVID is clinically diagnosed and cannot be definitively diagnosed independently with the use of blood work, imaging, or any other testing at this time. Some biomarkers, such as low blood cortisol in the morning, must be correlated to the symptoms. Long COVID is an actual condition; it is not imaginary in your mind, and it is not caused by anxiety, depression, or any other mental disorder.

Symptoms can be categorized by function or by anatomical body area. Here, I separate symptoms by functional organ system. As you go thru each of the cause's symptoms, you may notice a lot of similarities between the symptoms of each cause.

Here is an overview of the most common symptoms classified by organ system. These are the most common presentations, and this list is <u>not comprehensive</u>:

1. Respiratory System

- **Shortness of Breath:** Persistent difficulty breathing or a feeling of not getting adequate air, even with minimal exertion. This condition may be associated with *hypoxia* or low oxygen saturation observed on a pulse oximetry device.
- **Cough:** A chronic cough that can be dry or productive.

- **Chest Pain:** Discomfort or pain in the chest, which may be related to breathing issues.

2. Cardiovascular System

- **Palpitations:** Sensations of rapid, fluttering, or pounding heartbeats.
- **Chest Pain:** This pain can also be associated with cardiovascular issues and may require cardiological evaluation.
- **Postural Orthostatic Tachycardia Syndrome (POTS):** It is a condition that impacts heart rate and Blood Pressure (BP), causing dizziness and fainting upon standing.
- **Chest tightness**
- **Inappropriate Sinus Tachycardia:** fast heart rate.

3. Neurological System

- **Cognitive Impairment ("Brain Fog"):** In this case, the patient endures issues with memory, attention, and executive function.
- **Headaches:** Persistent or recurring headaches.
- **Dizziness and Balance Problems:** Feelings of lightheadedness or unsteadiness, increasing the risk of falls.
- **Peripheral Neuropathy** causes numbness, tingling, or pain in the hands and feet.
- **Vibrations in the chest or any part of the body**
- **Insomnia** – lack or absence of deep sleep prominence of sympathetic nervous system overdrive.
- **Fatigue**
- **Hoarseness, vocal cord dysfunction**
- **Neuropathies, including small fiber neuropathy**

4. Musculoskeletal System

- **Joint and Muscle Pain**: Continuous aches and pains in joints and muscles, often exacerbated by physical activity.
- **Muscle Weakness:** Reduced strength and endurance, affecting mobility.

5. Gastrointestinal System

- **Diarrhea:** Persistent or intermittent loose stools.
- **Nausea:** A feeling of sickness or discomfort in the stomach.
- **Abdominal Pain**: Ongoing pain or discomfort in the abdominal area.
- **Heartburn (GERD)**
- **Changes in stool color**
- **Gastroparesis**
- **Dysphagia (painful or trouble swallowing)**

6. Dermatological System

- **Skin Rashes:** Various types of rashes or changes in skin texture.
- **Hair Loss:** Increased hair shedding or thinning, referred to as telogen effluvium.

7. Endocrine System

- **New-onset Diabetes or Worsening of Pre-existing Diabetes:** Changes in blood sugar levels and insulin sensitivity.
- **Thyroid Dysfunction:** Abnormal thyroid function tests and symptoms of hypo- or hyperthyroidism.
- **Changes in the regularity of periods, early onset menopause**

8. Psychological and Psychiatric Symptoms

- **Depression:** Persistent feelings of grief or hopelessness.
- **Anxiety:** Ongoing feelings of worry or fear.
- **Post-Traumatic Stress Disorder (PTSD):** Psychological distress following the trauma of severe illness.
- **Derealization**
- **Depersonalization**

9. Hematologic System

- **Blood Clots:** Increased risk of developing blood clots, leading to conditions such as Deep Vein Thrombosis (DVT) or Pulmonary Embolism (PE).

10. Renal System

- **Kidney Dysfunction:** Evidence of impaired kidney function may be detected through laboratory tests.
- **Kidney stones**

11. Immune System

- **Persistent Inflammation:** Ongoing low-grade inflammation can affect multiple organ systems.
- **Autoimmune Reactions:** Developing new autoimmune conditions or exacerbation of existing ones.

12. Otolaryngological System (ENT)

- **Loss of Taste and Smell (anosmia and ageusia):** Partial or complete loss of taste (ageusia) and smell (anosmia), persisting for months.
- **Abnormal taste and smell (parosmia and dysgeusia)** can be pleasant or unpleasant.

- **Phantosmia** is a smell hallucination where you smell something that is not there.
- Ear pressure/ear fullness/Eustachian tube dysfunction

13. Eyes

Vision changes can be a symptom of Long COVID, affecting people even after they recover from the initial infection. Some of the common vision-related issues reported include:

1. Blurry Vision

- Some Long COVID patients experience difficulty focusing or have blurred vision, which can come and go or be persistent.

2. Eye Pain or Discomfort

- Patients may feel pain or discomfort in or around the eyes, often linked to headaches or light sensitivity.

3. Dry Eyes

- Long COVID may cause dry eyes, where the eyes feel gritty or uncomfortable due to reduced tear production.

4. Light Sensitivity (Photophobia)

- Increased sensitivity to light, also known as photophobia, is commonly reported. This can make it uncomfortable to be in bright environments.

5. Floaters

- Some individuals experience an increase in "floaters," small shapes or spots that drift across the field of vision.

6. Double Vision

- Some patients report seeing double or having trouble with depth perception.

Causes of eye problems

- **Inflammation**: COVID-19 can cause inflammation throughout the body, including in the eyes. This may affect the optic nerve or other parts of the visual system.
- **Vascular Issues**: COVID-19 can impact blood vessels, potentially affecting blood flow to the eyes and leading to vision problems.
- **Neurological Impact**: Since COVID-19 affects the nervous system, including the brain, it can disrupt the signals that control vision.

14. Reproductive System

- **Menstrual Irregularities:** Changes in menstrual cycle regularity, flow, or symptoms.
- Early onset menopause

15. Whole Body

- Post-exertional malaise
- Exercise intolerance
- Chronic fatigue

16.Head, Eyes, Nose, Mouth

- Dry eyes
- Dry mouth
- Burning mouth syndrome
- COVID tongue
- Pressure headache
- Face pressure
- Head pressure
- Trigeminal neuralgia
- Hair loss

It is essential to know that not everyone will have every one of these symptoms, and that may be due to which cause is the most prominent. Long COVID has many different presentations, which makes it challenging to diagnose. Patients with Long COVID typically have 15-18 symptoms.

References:

1. Batiha, G.ES., Al-kuraishy, H.M., Al-Gareeb, A.I. *et al.* Pathophysiology of Post-COVID syndromes: a new perspective. *Virol J* **19**, 158 (2022).

   https://DOI.org/10.1186/s12985-022-01891-2

2. Davis, H. E., Assaf, G. S., McCorkell, L., Wei, H., Low, R. J., Re'im, Y., et al. (2021). Characterizing Long COVID in an international cohort: 7 months of symptoms and their impact. EClinicalMedicine, 38, 101019.

   https://DOI.org/10.1016/j.eclinm.2021.101019

3. Hayes LD, Ingram J, Sculthorpe NF. More Than 100 Persistent Symptoms of SARS-CoV-2 (Long COVID): A Scoping Review. Front Med (Lausanne). 2021 Nov 1;8:750378. DOI: 10.3389/fmed.2021.750378. PMID: 34790680; PMCID: PMC8591053.

Post-Exertional Malaise (PEM)

Post-exertional Malaise (PEM) is a hallmark symptom of Long COVID and also other conditions like Myalgic Encephalomyelitis/Chronic Fatigue Syndrome/ (ME/CFS). PEM is characterized by a significant deterioration of symptoms following physical, mental, or emotional exertion. The exhaustion felt is way out of proportion to the exertion in terms of how severe or how long it lasts. PEM may be caused by multiple conditions, including chronic inflammation, metabolic dysregulation, hormone imbalance, oxidative stress, mitochondrial dysfunction, non-restorative sleep, or dysautonomia.

Possible Causes of PEM in Long COVID

1. **Immune System Dysfunction** - Long COVID may involve ongoing, low-level inflammation both in the body and brain, which can be exacerbated by exertion, leading to an overactive immune response and PEM. A leaky blood-brain barrier can contribute to the neuroinflammation.

2. **Autonomic Nervous System (ANS) Dysfunction**

   - **Dysautonomia:** Many Long COVID patients experience dysautonomia, which impacts the regulation of autonomic functions such as heart rate and BP. Exertion can exacerbate these dysregulations, leading to PEM.

   - **POTS:** Postural Orthostatic Tachycardia Syndrome (POTS)—a form of dysautonomia—is common in Long COVID and can lead to symptoms such as fatigue and dizziness after minimal exertion.

3. Mitochondrial Dysfunction – Lowered energy production. Mitochondria are responsible for producing energy in cells. In Long COVID, mitochondrial dysfunction may impair energy production, leading to an energy deficit after exertion and contributing to PEM.

- **Oxidative Stress - Increased** oxidative stress can damage cells and tissues, leading to fatigue and other symptoms. Likewise, exertion can enhance oxidative stress, triggering PEM.

4. Metabolic Dysregulation / Metabolic Syndrome - Altered metabolism of fatty acids and glucose in Long COVID, leading to an inability to sustain physical or mental activity without triggering PEM.

5. Hormonal Imbalance - Dysregulation of the Hypothalamic-Pituitary-Adrenal (HPA) axis in Long COVID can contribute to PEM by impairing the body's ability to manage stress and recover from exertion.

7. Muscle Abnormalities - Muscle inflammation and damage can increase fatigue and pain after exertion, contributing to PEM.

8. Non-Restorative Sleep - Long COVID patients often experience sleep disturbances, impairing recovery and exacerbating symptoms after exertion.

In general, managing PEM in Long COVID typically involves activity management (such as **pacing**), lifestyle modifications, and treating the symptoms. Treating symptoms is fine in the short term, but I propose treating the causes instead. I primarily target dysautonomia and mitochondrial dysfunction, which you can find in the treatment of causes section below. Under mitochondrial dysfunction, my goals are to minimize oxidative stress, induce mitophagy and autophagy of damaged cells, and promote new mitochondria biogenesis. Furthermore, I focus on reducing the sympathetic nervous system or fight or flight influence under dysautonomia treatments while increasing the vagus nerve influence.

Shortness of Breath (SOB) or Dyspnea

Shortness of breath, or dyspnea, is a common symptom experienced by individuals with Long COVID. The causes of this symptom are multifaceted and involve multiple body systems. I first determine if the SOB is associated with a low oxygen saturation, which can be measured using a pulse oximeter. If so, I want to rule out lung or heart involvement first. If it is not, I consider dysautonomia and mitochondrial dysfunction as causes. Exertional SOB is more common than resting SOB in Long COVID. Resting SOB is more concerning.

While lung fibrosis and heart damage are considered a rare cause, if you were on a ventilator, have preexisting lung or heart disease, or are experiencing hypoxia (low oxygen saturation), these still must be ruled out as a cause of your SOB with a chest x-ray, chest CT, chest MRI, or an echocardiogram. Moreover, pulmonary function tests may be needed to evaluate lung function and capacity. A cardiac stress test may be considered if chest pain associated with the SOB occurs to look at angina. Shortness of breath after meals may be related to **excess histamine**.

1. Lung

- **Lung Fibrosis:** Long COVID can cause scarring (fibrosis) of the lung tissue, which impairs gas exchange and decreases lung function.
- **Interstitial Lung Disease:** Inflammation and damage to the lung tissue can result in chronic respiratory issues, leading to persistent shortness of breath.
- **Persistent Lung Inflammation** - Continued lung inflammation can cause swelling and damage to the airways, reducing airflow and leading to breathlessness.

- **Viral Persistence** - In some cases, remnants of the virus may remain in the body, causing ongoing symptoms, including shortness of breath.
- **Blood Clots** in the lungs (pulmonary microthrombi) or larger pulmonary emboli can obstruct blood flow and cause breathing issues. These can be screened for with a blood D-dimer test.

2. Heart

- **Cardiomyopathy**
- **Myocarditis** - COVID-19 can lead to inflammation of the heart muscle (myocarditis), impairing the heart's ability to pump blood effectively, resulting in shortness of breath.
- **Pericarditis**

3. Dysautonomia/POTS

- Some Long COVID patients develop POTS, leading to an abnormally high heart rate and shortness of breath upon standing.
- **Autonomic Nervous System Dysfunction:** Damage or dysregulation of the autonomic nervous system can influence respiratory regulation, causing shortness of breath.

4. Central Nervous System

COVID-19 can affect the brain and brainstem, impacting the control of respiration and leading to breathing issues.

5. Muscle Weakness or pain

- **Deconditioning:** Prolonged illness and inactivity can lead to muscle weakness, including the respiratory muscles, contributing to shortness of breath. Moreover, myalgias in the chest wall can also do this.
- **Mitochondrial Dysfunction**

I focus on treating the cause, which oftentimes is mitochondrial dysfunction. **Remember that severe or complete mitochondrial dysfunction can cause organ failure and death. Take this aspect of Long COVID seriously.**

Brain fog

What are executive functions of the brain? These functions start to develop in teenagers and are controlled by the prefrontal cortex in the brain.

1. **Working Memory**: The ability to hold and manipulate information in your mind for short periods. For example, remembering a phone number long enough to dial it.
2. **Cognitive Flexibility**: The capacity to switch between thinking about different ideas or adapting to new situations. This helps in problem-solving when plans change.
3. **Inhibitory Control**: The ability to suppress impulsive responses or distractions to stay focused on tasks. This includes resisting the urge to interrupt others or give in to temptations.
4. **Planning and Organization**: The skill of setting goals, developing steps to achieve them, and arranging tasks in a logical order.
5. **Emotional Regulation**: The ability to manage emotions and behaviors effectively, particularly in stressful situations.

Other Brain Fog Symptoms:

- feeling as if your head is in the clouds
- loss of executive functions
- lessened concentration ability
- losing your train of thought
- mental exhaustion

- not delivering the right words during the speech
- confusion
- challenges processing information
- issues with paying attention
- feeling disoriented
- slow thought process and reaction time
- memory problems

The exact mechanisms behind brain fog in Long COVID are not thoroughly studied, but several potential causes have been specified:

- **Dysautonomia:** Some Long COVID patients experience dysautonomia, a condition where the Autonomic Nervous System (ANS) is impaired. It can affect heart rate, BP, and brain function, contributing to brain fog symptoms.

- **Leaky blood-brain barrier-** The virus can disrupt the integrity of the blood-brain barrier, allowing detrimental substances to enter the brain and cause inflammation and damage.

- **Mitochondrial dysfunction** – neurons are energy dependent.

- **Unrefreshing Sleep –** this effect is cumulative. Your brain requires adequate rest to reset for the next day.

- **Reduced Oxygen Supply:** COVID-19 can impact the respiratory system and reduce oxygen levels in the blood, leading to hypoxia (low oxygen supply). More significantly, chronic hypoxia can impair brain function and lead to cognitive deficits.

My treatment objectives for brain fog are to minimize neuroinflammation, restore normal blood flow, and correct dysautonomia to allow for restorative sleep. I do not rely on stimulants like those utilized for ADHD, caffeine, or nicotine.

Chest Pain

Once you have ruled out cardiac and pulmonary causes such as pericarditis and myocarditis, in Long COVID, chest pain can be neuropathic, from reactivation of chicken pox zoster virus, costochondritis, muscle strain, or acid reflux.

Cardiac Causes

1. **Angina**: Chest pain due to reduced blood flow to the heart muscle, often triggered by physical exertion or stress.
2. **Myocardial Infarction (Heart Attack)**: A blockage in one or more coronary arteries leads to heart muscle damage.
3. **Pericarditis**: Inflammation of the pericardium, the sac surrounding the heart, causing sharp, pleuritic chest pain.
4. **Myocarditis**: Inflammation of the heart muscle, which can cause chest pain, fatigue, and irregular heartbeats.
5. **Aortic Dissection**: It is a tear in the inner layer of the aorta, causing severe, ripping chest pain that radiates to the back.

Pulmonary Causes

1. **Pulmonary Embolism**: It is due to a blood clot in the lung arteries migrating from a deep vein thrombosis (DVT) from the legs), causing sudden, sharp chest pain, shortness of breath, and possibly hemoptysis.
2. **Pneumothorax**: Air in the pleural space, leading to sudden, sharp chest pain and difficulty breathing.

3. **Pneumonia**: Lung infection causing pleuritic chest pain, fever, and cough.
4. **Pleuritis (Pleurisy)**: Inflammation of the pleura, the membranes surrounding the lungs, leading to sharp chest pain that aggravates with breathing or coughing.

Gastrointestinal Causes

1. **Gastroesophageal Reflux Disease (GERD)**: Acid reflux from the stomach into the esophagus causes a burning chest pain, which is also called *heartburn*.
2. **Esophageal Spasm**: Abnormal contractions of the esophagus cause intense chest pain, often confused with cardiac pain.
3. **Peptic Ulcer**: Ulcers in the stomach or duodenum can develop burning or gnawing pain, sometimes felt in the chest.

Musculoskeletal Causes

1. **Costochondritis**: Inflammation of the cartilage connecting the ribs to the sternum, causing localized chest pain that can be reproduced by pressing the chest.
2. **Muscle Strain**: Overuse or injury to the chest muscles can cause localized pain that worsens with movement.

Psychological Causes

1. **Anxiety and Panic Attacks**: Can cause chest pain or discomfort, often accompanied by rapid heartbeat, sweating, and shortness of breath.

Other Causes of chest pain

1. **Herpes Zoster (Shingles)**: Reactivation of the chickenpox virus causes a painful rash and chest pain along the affected nerve.

2. **Thoracic Outlet Syndrome**: Compression of nerves or blood vessels between the collarbone and first rib can cause chest and shoulder pain.

Neuropathies

What are neuropathies? They are an abnormal nerve response from damage or irritation to the **peripheral nervous system** (all of the nerves outside the brain and spinal cord), which connects the brain and spinal cord to the rest of the body. Irritation is technically called neuritis, but it is the same idea. Neuropathy can affect sensory, motor, or autonomic nerves, leading to symptoms like numbness, tingling, weakness, or pain. Neuropathies cannot occur in the brain or spinal cord because both are part of the central nervous system.

Long COVID can affect any nerve in the body. An irritated nerve causes tingling, numbness, pins and needles (paresthesia), pain (shooting, burning, electrical), and sometimes weakness. It can be intermittent. Neuritis and neuropathies can involve any nerve. If it affects the sciatic nerve, it is called *sciatica*. If it involves the trigeminal nerve, it is called *trigeminal neuralgia*.

Neuropathies and **Neuritis** can present in several different ways depending on what the nerve or nerves control or do:

1. **Pain** – the most common result of neuropathy is simply pain. The pain tends to be burning and sharp. It is often associated with numbness or tingling. The pain doesn't change if you squeeze or massage the tender spot. Some report a sensation of ants crawling on your skin.

2. **Internal vibrations / body vibrations** – my opinion is that this is also a type of neuritis or neuropathy.

3. Dysautonomia is also known as **autonomic neuropathy**.

4. **Tinnitus** – in my opinion, a neuropathy or neuritis is responsible for tinnitus in Long COVID. The irritation can come from dysautonomia or from chronic inflammation. Some people respond immediately after a stellate ganglion procedure or EAT suggesting that dysautonomia is responsible for this.

Common Causes of Neuropathy

1. **Diabetes** (Diabetic Neuropathy) – The most common cause, leading to nerve damage from high blood sugar.

2. **Autoimmune Disorders** – Conditions like lupus, rheumatoid arthritis, and Guillain-Barré syndrome can cause the immune system to attack the nerves.

3. **Infections** – Viruses such as HIV, shingles, Lyme disease, and even COVID-19 can trigger nerve damage.

4. **Toxins** – Exposure to heavy metals or certain medications can damage nerves. I know, I know, but trust me, this is a rare cause.

5. **Physical Trauma** – Injuries from accidents or repetitive stress can compress nerves.

6. **Nutritional Deficiencies** – Lack of vitamins like B12, B6, and folate (B9) can cause nerve damage or nerve dysfunction.

Neuropathy in the Context of Long COVID

Long COVID is associated with various neurological symptoms, including **neuropathy**, which may arise due to several mechanisms:

1. **Immune-Mediated Nerve Damage** - Long COVID can trigger an autoimmune response, where the body's immune system mistakenly attacks healthy nerves, leading to conditions like **small fiber neuropathy** (SFN). SFN is a type of neuropathy that affects

small sensory fibers, leading to burning pain, numbness, and tingling.

2. **Inflammation and Cytokine Release** - The inflammatory response caused by SARS-CoV-2 can lead to nerve damage. Persistent **systemic inflammation** and elevated cytokines can contribute to nerve injury and dysfunction, which manifests as chronic pain or sensory abnormalities.

3. **Microvascular Damage** - Long COVID has been linked to **microvascular dysfunction**, which can impair blood supply to nerves, leading to **ischemic injury** of peripheral nerves and neuropathic symptoms.

4. **Direct Viral Invasion** - In some cases, the virus may directly infect nerve tissues, contributing to neuropathy.

5. **Dysautonomia -** Long COVID has also been linked to autonomic dysfunction, which affects the autonomic nerves controlling involuntary functions like heart rate and digestion. Dysautonomia often presents alongside neuropathic symptoms, especially in Long COVID patients with **Postural Orthostatic Tachycardia Syndrome (POTS)**.

Clinical Evidence

Studies have shown that a subset of Long COVID patients develop **peripheral neuropathy** due to immune-mediated mechanisms or ongoing inflammation. For example, research has linked **small fiber neuropathy** and autonomic neuropathies with Long COVID, which may result in long-lasting sensory and autonomic disturbances.

Small fiber neuropathy (SFN)

Effects the nerve endings often in your feet and sometimes your hands. It affects the **small sensory nerve fibers** responsible for transmitting pain, temperature, and autonomic signals. These fibers are part of the peripheral nervous system and are essential for functions like sensation and autonomic regulation (e.g., heart rate, blood pressure, and sweating). Damage to these fibers can lead to **pain**, **burning sensations**, **tingling**, **numbness**, and autonomic dysfunction. SFN may also contribute to **dysautonomia**. The most common type is diabetic neuropathy. There is some evidence that **IVIG** (intravenous immunoglobulin therapy) can be helpful in this case.

Small fiber neuropathy (SFN) is a type of peripheral neuropathy that primarily affects the small nerve fibers in the peripheral nervous system. These fibers include unmyelinated C fibers and thinly myelinated A-delta fibers, which are responsible for transmitting pain, temperature, and autonomic functions. Symptoms usually start in the distal extremities (hands and feet) and can progress proximally. Small fiber neuropathy is a confounding disease and is associated with various medical health conditions. In 50% of cases, the cause of SFN is identified, while in many cases, the cause of SFN is unknown (idiopathic), which makes the treatment process more complex. SFN has been linked to both ME/CFS and POTS.

Symptoms

- **Pain**: Often described as burning, shooting, or stabbing sensations, typically in the hands and feet.

- **Temperature Sensitivity**: Patients may experience altered sensations to hot or cold stimuli.
- **Skin color changes**
- **Numbness**: Loss of feeling or a "pins and needles" sensation, especially in the extremities.
- **Autonomic Dysfunction**: Symptoms can include abnormal sweating, changes in blood pressure, and gastrointestinal issues.
- **Bladder and bowel problems**
- include distal, symmetric burning pain, allodynia, impaired temperature sensation, paresthesias, and numbness.
- Negative nerve conduction tests and EMG results

Diagnosis

- **Clinical Evaluation**: A thorough history and physical examination to assess symptoms.
- **Quantitative Sensory Testing (QST)**: Measures sensory thresholds for pain, temperature, and touch.
- **Skin Biopsy**: A definitive test that examines small nerve fibers in the skin. A reduction in the density of these fibers supports the diagnosis of SFN.
- **Anti-TS-HDS** and **anti-FGFR-3 antibodies**, are seen in 20%–50% of SFN cases and dysautonomia.

Exclude all other conditions and reasons that cause neuropathies

1. Diabetes

- Diabetic neuropathy
- Glucose intolerance

2. Infections

- Viral: HIV, herpes zoster, cytomegalovirus (CMV)
- Bacterial: Lyme disease, leprosy

3. Autoimmune Disorders *

- Guillain-Barré syndrome
- Systemic Lupus
- Rheumatoid arthritis
- Sjögren's syndrome
- Sarcoidosis
- Celiac disease

4. Genetic Disorders

- Hereditary neuropathies (e.g., Charcot-Marie-Tooth disease)
- Genetic mutations affecting nerve function

5. Toxins

- Alcohol (ethanol), also leads to Vitamin B12 deficiency.
- Heavy metals (lead, mercury)
- Certain medications (chemotherapy agents)

6. Nutritional Deficiencies

- Vitamin B12 deficiency
- Vitamin B1 (thiamine) deficiency
- Vitamin B6 toxicity

7. Trauma or Injury

- Compression or entrapment (e.g., carpal tunnel syndrome)
- Direct nerve injury

8. Systemic Diseases

- Chronic kidney disease
- Liver disease
- Thyroid disorders

9. Vascular Disorders

- Peripheral artery disease
- Vasculitis

10. Metabolic Disorders

- Metabolic syndrome
- Hypothyroidism

11. Inflammatory Disorders

- Inflammatory demyelinating polyneuropathy

12. Tumors

- Tumors compressing nerves (benign or malignant)

13. Idiopathic

- In many cases, the cause of neuropathy remains unknown.

14. Other Conditions

- Multiple sclerosis
- Amyloidosis

15. Medications

- **Chemotherapy Agents**
  - **Vincristine**: Commonly used for cancer treatment, can cause peripheral neuropathy.
  - **Paclitaxel**: Another chemotherapy drug associated with neuropathic pain.
  - **Cisplatin**: Known to cause peripheral nerve damage.
- **Antiretroviral Drugs**
  - **Zidovudine (AZT)**: Used in HIV treatment, associated with neuropathy.
  - **Didanosine (ddI)**: Can cause peripheral neuropathy.

- **Antibiotics**
  - **Metronidazole**: High doses or prolonged use may lead to neuropathy.
  - **Fluoroquinolones**: Such as ciprofloxacin; rare cases of peripheral neuropathy reported.
- **Anticonvulsants**
  - **Phenytoin**: Used for seizure disorders, can lead to neuropathy with prolonged use.
  - **Carbamazepine**: Associated with peripheral neuropathy.
- **Antiarrhythmics (medications to stop heart arrythmias)**
  - **Lidocaine:** High doses or prolonged use can lead to peripheral neuropathy or other neurological effects, including tingling and numbness.
  - **Disopyramide:** anticholinergic effects that may lead to peripheral neuropathy symptoms.
  - **Quinidine**
  - **Procainamide:** neuropathy, particularly with long-term use.
  - **Sotalol:** rare reports of peripheral neuropathy, often in patients receiving high doses or prolonged therapy.
  - **Flecainide**: neurological side effects, including neuropathy, may occur in some patients.
- **Immunosuppressants**
  - **Cyclosporine**: Used in organ transplantation; may cause peripheral neuropathy.
- **Cholesterol-Lowering Drugs**
  - **Statins**: Some reports suggest a link between statin use and neuropathy, though evidence is mixed.
- **Heavy Metals and Industrial Chemicals**

    - **Lead toxicity**
    - **Mercury toxicity**
- **Antidepressants**
    - **Amitriptyline**: Can cause neuropathic symptoms, especially at higher doses.
- **Other Medications**
    - **Metformin**: While not directly causing neuropathy, it **can lead to vitamin B12 deficiency**, which is associated with neuropathy.
    - **Bortezomib**: Used for multiple myeloma, can lead to peripheral neuropathy.

IVIG

Intravenous immunoglobulin (IVIG) is being explored as a treatment option for Long COVID patients experiencing SFN, particularly when an autoimmune component is suspected. While research is still evolving, treatment protocols are being adapted from existing guidelines for autoimmune SFN.

Mechanisms of IVIG in Long COVID SFN

In Long COVID-associated SFN, IVIG is thought to work by:

- **Modulating autoantibodies**: IVIG can neutralize harmful autoantibodies that may attack small nerve fibers.
- **Reducing inflammation**: IVIG reduces complement-mediated inflammation, which can play a role in nerve damage.
- **Regulating immune function**: IVIG has immunomodulatory effects that help balance an overactive immune response, a feature in many autoimmune conditions.
- **Promoting nerve regeneration**: By controlling inflammation and autoimmunity, IVIG may create an environment conducive to the regeneration of damaged small nerve fibers.

IVIG Protocols for Long COVID-Related SFN

1. Initial IVIG Dose

- Patients typically receive an initial high dose of IVIG to address the acute phase of inflammation and immune dysregulation.

- A common starting dose is **2g/kg**, administered over **2–5 consecutive days**.
- Hydration before and during the infusion is recommended to reduce the risk of side effects, such as headaches and aseptic meningitis.

2. Maintenance Therapy

- Following the initial dose, **maintenance infusions** are often required to sustain the therapeutic effect.
- A typical maintenance dose is **0.4g/kg** administered every **3–4 weeks**, depending on the patient's response and the severity of symptoms.
- The duration of maintenance therapy can vary, with some patients requiring several months of treatment, while others may benefit from long-term therapy.

3. Monitoring and Adjustment

- Patients should be closely monitored for both clinical improvement and potential side effects, such as headache, renal dysfunction, and rare immune reactions.
- The infusion rate and dosage may be adjusted based on the individual's tolerance and therapeutic response.

Evidence of IVIG for Long COVID SFN

Although specific studies on IVIG for Long COVID-related SFN are still emerging, existing case reports and studies on autoimmune SFN support the use of IVIG in similar post-viral neuropathies:

- **Case Reports**: Some patients with Long COVID and SFN have shown improvement in symptoms such as neuropathic pain, fatigue, and autonomic dysfunction following IVIG therapy. These improvements are consistent with findings in other autoimmune and post-viral SFN cases.

- **Comparative Studies**: Studies on other autoimmune conditions like **Sjögren's syndrome** and **sarcoidosis** with SFN have shown that IVIG can reduce neuropathic pain and improve quality of life, suggesting that similar benefits may be possible for Long COVID patients.

IVIG Treatment Considerations in Long COVID

1. **Patient Selection**: IVIG is generally reserved for Long COVID patients with confirmed SFN and suspected autoimmune involvement. Diagnostic tests such as skin biopsies or nerve conduction studies can help confirm SFN.

2. **Risk Factors**: Special care is taken for individuals with underlying kidney disease, advanced age, or clotting disorders, as IVIG can increase the risk of renal dysfunction and thrombotic events. Hydration and slow infusion rates are critical to minimizing these risks.

3. **Symptom Management**: IVIG is part of a broader treatment plan, which may include medications for pain relief (e.g., gabapentin, pregabalin), physical therapy, and lifestyle modifications like diet and exercise.

Common Side Effects

- Headache
- Fever
- Joint pain
- Chest pain
- Vomiting
- Nausea

- Fatigue
- Dizziness
- Chills
- Rash (less common)
- Fluid overload

Rare Side Effects

Though uncommon, serious side effects of IVIG have been reported, including:

- **Aseptic meningitis**: Inflammation of the membranes around the brain and spinal cord can cause severe headaches, usually appearing within 72 hours after infusion. Those with a history of migraines may be more prone to this. Staying well-hydrated before IVIG can help reduce this risk. It's important to contact a healthcare provider if a severe headache occurs, especially if it doesn't improve with acetaminophen or ibuprofen. However, not all post-infusion headaches indicate aseptic meningitis.

- **Heart attack, stroke, and deep vein thrombosis (DVT)**: IVIG has been linked to blood clots that can cause these serious conditions. This risk may be related to an enzyme contaminant, factor XIa, found in some plasma preparations. Manufacturers now test for and remove this enzyme to reduce risk. People with risk factors like heart disease, clotting disorders, hypertension, diabetes, high cholesterol, kidney disease, advanced age, obesity, or immobility should take precautions, including proper hydration and avoiding exceeding the recommended infusion rate.

- **Kidney dysfunction or failure**: While acute kidney failure has been seen following IVIG infusions, does not respond to standard pain relievers like acetaminophen or ibuprofen, as it may indicate aseptic meningitis.

- **Heart attack and stroke**: IVIG infusions have been linked to a higher risk of **blood clots**, which can lead to heart attacks, strokes, or **pulmonary embolism** (a blockage in the lungs). The risk is thought to be due to a contaminant in plasma preparations called **factor XIa**, which manufacturers now test for and remove. People with risk factors such as heart disease, advanced age, a history of blood clots, high blood pressure, diabetes, high cholesterol, kidney disease, obesity, or immobility may be more vulnerable. Staying hydrated and keeping the infusion rate within recommended limits is crucial to minimize this risk.

- **Acute kidney failure**: IVIG has been associated with **acute renal (kidney) failure**, especially in people over 65 or those with pre-existing kidney issues. The risk is greatly reduced since **sucrose-based IVIG products**, which were responsible for most cases, are no longer in use.

- **Anaphylaxis**: A severe allergic reaction known as **anaphylaxis** is very rare and may occur in people with **IgA deficiency** who have developed IgE antibodies against human IgA. However, this connection is still controversial, and no tests are currently available for these antibodies. Newer IVIG formulations have very low IgA concentrations, and subcutaneous immunoglobulin (SCIG) does not cause these reactions, making it a safer option for individuals with IgA-related concerns.

- **Hemolytic anemia**: In rare cases, IVIG can lead to **hemolytic anemia**, where the immune system destroys red blood cells, causing low blood counts. This is more likely to occur in people receiving high doses of IVIG for **autoimmune disorders** rather than those receiving it as replacement therapy.

In summary, while IVIG therapy is generally safe, it's important to monitor for these side effects, especially in individuals with pre-existing health conditions. Staying hydrated, following recommended infusion rates, and consulting a healthcare provider if symptoms arise can help minimize risks.

References:

- McAlpine, L., Zubair, A. S., Joseph, P., & Spudich, S. (2024). Case-control study of individuals with small fiber neuropathy after COVID-19. *Neurology® Neuroimmunology & Neuroinflammation*, 11(3). https://doi.org/10.1212/NXI.0000000000200244

- Geerts, M., de Greef, B. T. A., Sopacua, M., van Kuijk, S. M. J., Hoeijmakers, J. G. J., Faber, C. G., & Merkies, I. S. J. (2021). Intravenous immunoglobulin therapy in patients with painful idiopathic small fiber neuropathy. *Neurology*, 96(20), e2534-e2545. https://doi.org/10.1212/WNL.0000000000011919

- McAlpine, L. S., Zubair, A. S., Joseph, P., & Spudich, S. (2023). Small fiber neuropathy after COVID-19: A key to long COVID. *Preprint*. https://doi.org/10.1101/2023.11.07.23297764

- Manganotti P, Garascia G, Furlanis G, Stella AB. Efficacy of intravenous immunoglobulin (IVIg) on COVID-19-related neurological disorders over the last 2 years: an up-to-date narrative review. *Front Neurosci*;**17.** April 2023. DOI: 10.3389/fnins.2023.1159929

Gastroparesis

Gastroparesis is a condition characterized by delayed gastric emptying, where the stomach takes longer than normal to empty its contents into the small intestine. This leads to symptoms such as **nausea**, **vomiting**, **bloating**, **abdominal pain**, and feeling full quickly. In the context of **Long COVID**, gastroparesis can develop due to the effects of the SARS-CoV-2 virus on the **nervous system**, particularly the **vagus nerve**, which plays a crucial role in controlling the motility of the digestive tract.

- **Testing**
    - upper endoscopy
    - gastric emptying study
- **Dietary changes**
    - eat small and frequent meals
    - low fat
    - low fiber diet (fiber speeds transport)
    - pureed or liquid meals
- **Treatment**
    - prokinetic metoclopramide
    - antinausea medications like ondansetron
    - vagus nerve stimulation
    - Consider SGB and EAT

Tinnitus

In the article by Figueiredo et al. (2022), the authors explore the characteristics and potential causes of **tinnitus** emerging in the context of **COVID-19** and **Long COVID**. The study suggests that tinnitus associated with COVID-19 does not significantly differ in its presentation compared to tinnitus from other causes. While the presentation may not be different, the causes may certainly be. However, the article highlights several key mechanisms that could explain the onset of tinnitus in patients with Long COVID. About 8-30% of Long COVID sufferers also suffer from tinnitus depending on which study is quoted. Regardless, this still effects millions of people around the world and all from Long COVID. Tinnitus often occurs together with vertigo (room spinning) and dizziness (you are spinning).

1. Inflammation and Immune Activation

COVID-19 infection induces a significant **inflammatory response** and triggers **cytokine release** (cytokine storm) that can affect various body systems, including the auditory system. Inflammation around the **auditory nerve** or in the **cochlea** can contribute to tinnitus development. The prolonged inflammation seen in Long COVID may be a factor in the persistence of auditory symptoms.

2. Vascular Impairment

SARS-CoV-2 is known to cause **endothelial dysfunction** and vascular damage, which can impair blood flow to the cochlea and auditory structures. Reduced blood flow can lead to **cochlear ischemia**, which has been associated with hearing loss and tinnitus. This is consistent with the findings of Figueiredo et al. (2022), as vascular impairment due to COVID-19 may contribute to the onset of tinnitus.

3. Direct Viral Effects on the Auditory System

The presence of **ACE2 receptors** in the auditory pathway allows the virus to infect cells in the **inner ear** and related structures. The article suggests that direct viral invasion of these areas could alter normal auditory function, potentially leading to tinnitus. However, Figueiredo et al. (2022) emphasize that the characteristics of tinnitus associated with COVID-19 are similar to those caused by other conditions, indicating that this direct mechanism may not result in unique symptoms.

4. Stress and Psychological Factors

The pandemic has contributed to widespread stress, anxiety, and depression, which are known to exacerbate tinnitus. In Long COVID, ongoing physical symptoms and the uncertainty of recovery can further heighten stress levels, potentially worsening or sustaining tinnitus. Figueiredo et al. (2022) point out that psychological factors may play a significant role in the persistence of tinnitus in COVID-19 patients, as seen in other forms of tinnitus.

5. Neurological Involvement

COVID-19 can affect the **central nervous system** (CNS), including areas involved in auditory processing. This neurological impact, combined with peripheral auditory dysfunction, can lead to tinnitus. In their study, Figueiredo et al. (2022) discuss how both peripheral and central auditory pathways may be involved in the development of tinnitus in Long COVID.

6. Dysautonomia

I personally believe that Long COVID caused tinnitus is a form of dysautonomia induced neuritis. Irritation of the auditory nerve or the inner ear nerve endings. I have witnessed resolution of the tinnitus with SGB and with EAT procedures. I have seen improvement even with simple vagus nerve stimulation.

References:

1. Figueiredo, R. R., Penido, N. de O., Azevedo, A. A. de, Oliveira, P. M. de, Siqueira, A. G. de, Figueiredo, G. M. R. de, Schlee, W., & Langguth, B. (2022). Tinnitus emerging in the context of a COVID-19 infection seems not to differ in its characteristics from tinnitus unrelated to COVID-19. *Frontiers in Neurology*, 13, 974179. https://doi.org/10.3389/fneur.2022.974179

2. Wang D, Li P, Huang X, Liu Y, Mao S, Yin H, Wang N, Luo Y, Sun S. Exploring the Prevalence of Tinnitus and Ear-Related Symptoms in China After the COVID-19 Pandemic: Online Cross-Sectional Survey. JMIR Form Res. 2024 Apr 24;8:e54326. doi: 10.2196/54326. PMID: 38657236; PMCID: PMC11045005.

3. Geerts M, de Greef BTA, Sopacua M, van Kuijk SMJ, Hoeijmakers JGJ, Faber CG, Merkies ISJ. Intravenous Immunoglobulin Therapy in Patients With Painful Idiopathic Small Fiber Neuropathy. Neurology. 2021 May 18;96(20):e2534-e2545. doi: 10.1212/WNL.0000000000011919. Epub 2021 Mar 25. PMID: 33766992; PMCID: PMC8205474.

4. de Greef BT, Geerts M, Hoeijmakers JG, Faber CG, Merkies IS. Intravenous immunoglobulin therapy for small fiber neuropathy: study protocol for a randomized controlled trial. Trials. 2016 Jul 20;17(1):330. doi: 10.1186/s13063-016-1450-x. PMID: 27439408; PMCID: PMC4955261.

5. Manganotti P, Garascia G, Furlanis G, Buoite Stella A. Efficacy of intravenous immunoglobulin (IVIG) on COVID-19-related neurological disorders over the last 2 years: an up-to-date narrative review. Front Neurosci. 2023 Apr 25;17:1159929. doi: 10.3389/fnins.2023.1159929. PMID: 37179564; PMCID: PMC10166837.

6. Dalakas, M. C. (2024). Post-COVID Small Fiber Neuropathy, Implications of Innate Immunity, and Challenges on IVIG Therapy.

Neurology: Neuroimmunology & Neuroinflammation, 11(3). https://doi.org/10.1212/NXI.0000000000200248

7. McAlpine, L., Zubair, A. S., Joseph, P., & Spudich, S. (2024). Case-Control Study of Individuals With Small Fiber Neuropathy After COVID-19. *Neurology: Neuroimmunology & Neuroinflammation,* 11(3). https://doi.org/10.1212/NXI.0000000000200244

8. Levine, T. D. (2019). Small Fiber Neuropathy: Disease Classification Beyond Pain and Burning. *Journal of Central Nervous System Disease,* 11, 1179573519841794. https://doi.org/10.1177/1179573519841794

9. Camilleri, M. (2019). Gastroparesis: Etiology, clinical manifestations, and diagnosis. *UpToDate.* https://www.uptodate.com/contents/gastroparesis

Insomnia / Unrefreshed Sleep

Insomnia during Long COVID occurs due to several reasons. Insomnia can be due to trouble falling asleep or difficulty staying asleep. Both can cause unrefreshed sleep. What this means is that it doesn't matter how many actual hours you remain unconscious; it is how much and how much you spend in deep sleep. Deep sleep is where this magic happens. During this time, your body focuses on healing, regeneration, and maintenance. Have you noticed that cuts heal much faster overnight than during the day? Our bodies have limited resources. It needs to have a focus on where to prioritize its resources. During deep sleep, nearly everything is focused on your recovery. It is no wonder that if you don't get enough quality deep sleep (stage 3), you feel tired, grumpy, and sleepy even after waking up. Much of the brain fog and chronic fatigue can come from a lack of deep sleep.

To understand **insomnia,** you first have to understand what sleep is. We shift through various stages all night. Sleep is not spent in only one stage.

Stages of Sleep

- **Stage 1:** Lightest sleep, transition between wakefulness and sleep, slowed heartbeat, breathing, eye movements, and muscle relaxation with occasional twitches.

- **Stage 2:** Light sleep, further slowing of heart rate and breathing, cessation of eye movements, muscles relax more, and body temperature drops. Brain waves slow down.

- **Stage 3:** Deep or slow-wave sleep, marked by delta waves in the brain. It is the most restorative stage, with significant heart rate, breathing, and brain activity decreases. It is harder to wake someone from this stage.

- **REM Sleep:** Rapid eye movements, enhanced brain activity resembling wakefulness, vivid dreaming, temporary muscle paralysis (except for breathing and eye muscles), irregular breathing, and heart rate. It is essential for cognitive functions such as memory consolidation and mood regulation.

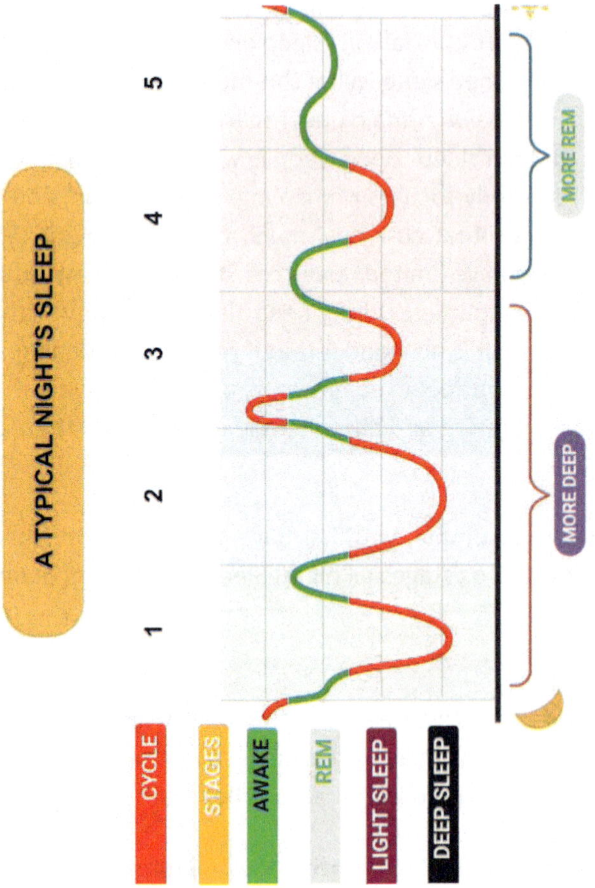

Chronic sleep deprivation or poor sleep quality can lead to multiple health issues, including cardiovascular diseases, obesity, diabetes, impaired immune function, mood disorders, and cognitive decline. Moreover, it will make everything associated with Long COVID worse.

Reasons for Unrefreshed Sleep

- Check for obstructive sleep apnea using a sleep study
- Check sleep hygiene and related habits
- Chronic inflammation
- Headaches
- Anxiety
- Pain
- Shortness of breath
- Dysautonomia

What to do about Unrefreshed Sleep

As much as I want to blame everything on Long COVID, we still need to look for horses first when we hear hoofbeats, not zebras. Typical stuff still happens commonly despite Long COVID. Unrefreshed sleep, where an individual wakes up tired and not well-rested despite seemingly adequate sleep duration, can be caused by various factors. It's not how long you stay unconscious; the quality of your sleep matters. First, look for non-Long COVID causes such as:

- Obstructive Sleep Apnea (OSA), do you snore? Not sure? Ask your bed partner! You can still have OSA without snoring, so a sleep study is needed to confirm.
- restless leg syndrome
- depression/anxiety
- fibromyalgia
- ME/CFS
- Discontinue nicotine patch
- Discontinue caffeine
- Discontinue alcohol

- **Sleep hygiene / Sleep habits**
    - Get natural daylight during the early part of the day especially before noon. Get sunlight exposure without any light barriers like windows or glasses.
    - Maintain regular physical activity if you are able and during the day not at night
    - Avoid long and late napping
    - Choose relaxing activities
    - Keep a regular bed time and wake up time even on weekends
    - Check the age of your mattress. Make sure mattress, pillow and blanket are comfortable.
    - Check the bedroom environment:
        - light pollution, especially blue light
        - Check the room temperature (Too hot? Too cold?)
        - Check the noise level
    - Avoid watching television, playing videos, playing games on your phone or computer, or eating in bed

If it is not caused by anything above, I next address the dysautonomia with the following:

- Vagus nerve stimulation
- Stellate ganglion block
- EAT procedure

Melatonin can help with circadian rhythm; it is not a sedative.

Antihistamines can help for short-term use only. If used every night, you will get used to antihistamines quickly, and it would not be as effective. These are meant to buy time rather than be a permanent solution.

Over-the-Counter (OTC) Options

1. Antihistamines

- Diphenhydramine (*e.g.,* Benadryl®)
- Doxylamine *(e.g.,* Unisom®)

2. Herbal Supplements

- Valerian root
- Chamomile
- Lavender

3. Natural Remedies

- Magnesium Supplements
- Glycine
- L-Theanine

Prescription Medications

1. Benzodiazepines – short-term use only due to their addictive nature.

- Temazepam (Restoril)
- Triazolam (Halcion)

2. Non-Benzodiazepine Sedative-Hypnotics

- Zolpidem (Ambien)
- Eszopiclone (Lunesta)
- Zaleplon (Sonata)

3. Orexin Receptor Antagonists

- Suvorexant (Belsomra®)
- Lemborexant (Dayvigo®)

4. Antidepressants

- Trazodone
- Mirtazapine (Remeron®)
- Doxepin (Silenor®)

References:

1. Moura, A. E. F., Oliveira, D. N., Torres, D. M., Tavares-Júnior, J. W. L., Nóbrega, P. R., Braga-Neto, P., & Sobreira-Neto, M. A. (2022). Central hypersomnia and chronic insomnia: Expanding the spectrum of sleep disorders in long COVID syndrome - A prospective cohort study. *BMC Neurology*, 22, 417. https://doi.org/10.1186/s12883-022-02950-3

2. Guezguez F, Romdhani M, Boutaleb-Joutei A, Chamari K, Ben Saad H. Management of long-COVID-19 patients with sleep disorders: practical advice to general practitioners. Libyan J Med. 2023 Dec;18(1):2182704. doi: 10.1080/19932820.2023.2182704. PMID: 36842064; PMCID: PMC9970199.

3. Tedjasukmana, R., Budikayanti, A., Islamiyah, W. R., Witjaksono, A. M. A. L., & Hakim, M. (2023). Sleep disturbance in post COVID-19 conditions: Prevalence and quality of life. *Frontiers in Neurology*, 13, 1095606. https://doi.org/10.3389/fneur.2022.1095606

4. Rauwerda, N. L., Kuut, T. A., Braamse, A. M. J., Csorba, I., Nieuwkerk, P., van Straten, A., & Knoop, H. (2024). Insomnia and sleep characteristics in post COVID-19 fatigue: A cross-sectional case-controlled study. *Journal of Psychosomatic Research*, 177, 111522. https://doi.org/10.1016/j.jpsychores.2023.111522

5. Hoang, H. T. X., Yeung, W. F., Truong, Q. T. M., Le, C. T., Bui, A. T. M., Bui, Q. V., & Le, Q. T. L. (2024). Sleep quality among non-hospitalized COVID-19 survivors: A national cross-sectional study. *Frontiers in Public Health*, 11, 1281012. https://doi.org/10.3389/fpubh.2023.1281012

Hair loss

Why do some have hair loss during Long COVID? In my opinion, there are two reasons:

1) Dysautonomia reduces blood flow to the scalp, slowing hair follicle growth

2) Hormonal imbalances between estrogen, progesterone, and testosterone.

The hair loss can often be reversed by applying GHK-Cu, a topical peptide. It increases blood flow and even reverses the dihydrotestosterone (DHT) influence on hair follicles of the scalp. You can apply red LED to the scalp for 30 minutes daily in the 625-650 nm range to accelerate the copper activity in the peptide.

GHK-Cu and Hair Loss

1. **Promotes Hair Growth**:
   - GHK-Cu has been shown to improve the health of hair follicles, stimulate the growth phase of the hair cycle (anagen phase), and increase hair thickness by regenerating hair follicles.
2. **Anti-Inflammatory Effects**:
   - Inflammation is linked to various forms of hair loss, such as androgenetic alopecia and alopecia areata. GHK-Cu helps by reducing pro-inflammatory cytokines, which can otherwise damage hair follicles.

3. **Improves Blood Flow and Nourishment**:
    - GHK-Cu can improve blood flow to the scalp, promoting the delivery of essential nutrients to hair follicles, which is crucial for hair growth.

4. **Antioxidant Activity**:
    - By neutralizing oxidative stress, which can contribute to hair follicle miniaturization and hair loss, GHK-Cu protects follicles from further damage.

References:

1. **Fischer, D. L., Wong, W. W., Rubin, M. G., & Frishberg, D. P. (1999).** "A 12-week study evaluating the efficacy of a copper tripeptide in promoting hair growth." *Journal of Investigative Dermatology*, 113(3), 416.

2. **Pickart, L., & Margolina, A. (2018).** "GHK and DNA: resetting the human genome to health." *BioEssays*, 40(5), 1700231.

3. **Pickart, L. (2008).** "The human tri-peptide GHK-Cu in plasma, a modulator of extracellular matrix, angiogenesis, and inflammation." *Journal of Biomaterials Science, Polymer Edition*, 19(8), 969-988.

Chest Pain

In the context of Long COVID, we must rule out myocarditis and pericarditis as the causes of chest pain. Without these causes, the other common causes are neuropathic, joint, as in costochondritis, and myalgia or muscle-caused pain.

Possible Causes of Chest Pain in Long COVID

1. **Cardiac Causes**

    - **Myocarditis**: Heart muscle inflammation can cause chest pain, fatigue, and palpitations.

    - **Pericarditis**: Inflammation of the pericardium can create sharp chest pain that may be exacerbated with deep breaths or lying down.

    - **Coronary Microvascular Dysfunction**: Even without major artery blockages, microvascular dysfunction can cause angina-like chest pain.

    - **Postural Orthostatic Tachycardia Syndrome (POTS)**: Can cause chest pain, palpitations, and dizziness upon standing.

2. **Pulmonary Causes**

    - **Pulmonary Embolism**: Blood clots in the lungs can cause sudden, sharp chest pain, shortness of breath, and hypoxia.

    - **Lung Fibrosis**: Persistent lung inflammation can lead to fibrotic variations and chest discomfort.

3. **Musculoskeletal Causes**

    - **Costochondritis**: Inflammation of the cartilage connecting ribs to the sternum can develop localized chest pain.
    - **Muscle Strain**: From coughing or physical activity.

4. **Gastrointestinal Causes**

    - **Gastroesophageal Reflux Disease (GERD)**: Can cause burning chest pain, which is often mistaken for cardiac pain.

References:

1. Collins RA, Ray N, Ratheal K, Colon A. Severe post-COVID-19 costochondritis in children. Proc (Bayl Univ Med Cent). 2021 Sep 27;35(1):56-57. doi: 10.1080/08998280.2021.1973274. PMID: 34966216; PMCID: PMC8477585.

2. Tan C, Lim R, Yeow M, Fong J, Balakrishnan T. Tietze's Syndrome Post-COVID-19 Infection in an Adult Patient. Cureus. 2022 Jul 31;14(7):e27499. doi: 10.7759/cureus.27499. PMID: 37817896; PMCID: PMC10564091.

3. Paruchuri SSH, Farwa UE, Jabeen S, Pamecha S, Shan Z, Parekh R, Lakkimsetti M, Alamin E, Sharma V, Haider S, Khan J, Razzaq W. Myocarditis and Myocardial Injury in Long COVID Syndrome: A Comprehensive Review of the Literature. Cureus. 2023 Jul 25;15(7):e42444. doi: 10.7759/cureus.42444. PMID: 37637608; PMCID: PMC10449234.

4. Dini FL, Baldini U, Bytyçi I, Pugliese NR, Bajraktari G, Henein MY. Acute pericarditis as a major clinical manifestation of long COVID-19 syndrome. Int J Cardiol. 2023 Mar 1;374:129-134. doi: 10.1016/j.ijcard.2022.12.019. Epub 2022 Dec 10. PMID: 36513284; PMCID: PMC9734068.

Metabolic Syndrome

Some people get a **metabolic syndrome** as part of Long COVID. It affects fatty acid metabolism, cholesterol, blood sugar levels, alcohol, and toxins. In general, it can cause:

- high blood pressure
- high fasting blood glucose
- weight gain
- high cholesterol and triglycerides

References:

1. Bai, F., et al. (2022). Mitochondrial dysfunction and metabolic syndrome in Long COVID patients. *Journal of Clinical Endocrinology & Metabolism*, 107(4), 1085-1092. https://doi.org/10.1210/clinem/dgac037

2. Montefusco, L., et al. (2021). Long-term impact of COVID-19 on glucose metabolism and diabetes. *Nature Metabolism*, 3(8), 792-800. https://doi.org/10.1038/s42255-021-00407-6

3. Rosenbaum, A. N., et al. (2022). Long-term effects of COVID-19 on metabolic health: Linking infection to insulin resistance and metabolic syndrome. *Diabetes Care*, 45(8), 1803-1812. https://doi.org/10.2337/dc22-0123

4. Menezes DC, Lima PDL, Lima IC, Uesugi JHE, Vasconcelos PFDC, Quaresma JAS, Falcão LFM. Metabolic Profile of Patients with Long COVID: A Cross-Sectional Study. Nutrients. 2023 Feb 27;15(5):1197. doi: 10.3390/nu15051197. PMID: 36904195; PMCID: PMC10005061.

Vestibular Symptoms in Long COVID

Vestibular problems have emerged as a significant issue in Long COVID, affecting patients' balance, spatial orientation, and overall quality of life. The vestibular system, located in the **inner ear**, is responsible for maintaining balance and coordinating movement, and damage to this system can lead to various symptoms. In Long COVID, vestibular dysfunction appears to be part of the broader neurological and autonomic dysregulation that some patients experience.

Symptoms

1. **Dizziness**: Patients frequently report feeling lightheaded or unsteady, particularly when standing or moving suddenly. This is one of the most common complaints.
2. **Vertigo**: Episodes of spinning sensation, where the patient feels as though their surroundings are moving or spinning around them, are reported. Vertigo in Long COVID can occur spontaneously or be triggered by certain movements, such as turning the head or standing up.
3. **Balance Issues**: Difficulty maintaining balance, particularly when walking, can lead to increased risk of falls. Patients may feel off-balance or unsteady, especially in low-light situations or when multitasking.
4. **Nausea and Motion Sickness**: Because the vestibular system helps coordinate movement and eye tracking, vestibular dysfunction can cause motion sickness or nausea, especially when moving quickly or riding in vehicles.

5. **Tinnitus and Hearing Changes**: In some cases, Long COVID patients with vestibular problems also report **tinnitus** (ringing in the ears) or hearing changes, possibly due to damage to the structures in the inner ear.
6. **Migraine-Like Symptoms**: In addition to vertigo, patients often report headache (which may be mild or severe), sensitivity to light (photophobia), sound (phonophobia), and nausea, all of which align with typical migraine symptoms.
7. **Cognitive and Fatigue-Related Symptoms**: Vestibular problems are often accompanied by **brain fog**, difficulty concentrating, and **fatigue**. The brain may struggle to compensate for the abnormal signals from the vestibular system, leading to mental exhaustion.

Potential Mechanisms of Vestibular Dysfunction

1. **Direct Viral Damage**: SARS-CoV-2 may directly invade the inner ear, including the vestibular system. Studies have suggested that the virus can cause inflammation or damage to the cochlea and vestibular nerves, leading to symptoms like vertigo and hearing loss.
2. **Inflammation and Immune Dysregulation**: COVID-19 often triggers a systemic inflammatory response, which can cause damage to neural structures, including the vestibular system. Persistent inflammation in Long COVID may exacerbate these issues over time.
3. **Autonomic Nervous System Dysregulation**: The autonomic nervous system, which controls involuntary functions like heart rate and blood pressure, is often dysregulated in Long COVID, leading to conditions like **Postural Orthostatic Tachycardia Syndrome (POTS)**. This dysregulation can affect blood flow to the brain and inner ear, contributing to dizziness, vertigo, and balance problems.
4. **Microvascular Damage**: COVID-19 can damage the small blood vessels, reducing blood flow to vital organs and tissues, including

the vestibular system. Reduced perfusion may lead to inadequate oxygen supply, resulting in vestibular symptoms.

5. **Neuroinflammation and Brainstem Dysfunction**: The brainstem, which coordinates balance and vestibular function, may be affected by COVID-related neuroinflammation. Dysfunction in this area could contribute to vestibular disturbances like dizziness and vertigo.

Management of Vestibular Dysfunction

- **Vestibular Rehabilitation Therapy (VRT)**: VRT includes exercises designed to improve balance, coordination, and gaze stabilization. It helps retrain the brain to compensate for vestibular dysfunction.
- **Medications**: Depending on symptoms, medications such as **meclizine** (for vertigo) or **beta blockers** (for POTS-related dizziness) may be used. However, long-term reliance on these medications is typically avoided.
- **Hydration and Blood Pressure Management**: For patients with autonomic dysfunction contributing to dizziness or lightheadedness, managing hydration, blood pressure, and heart rate may improve symptoms.
- **Lifestyle Modifications**: Patients may benefit from avoiding triggers (e.g., quick head movements or visual stimuli) and making adjustments in their environment to reduce fall risks.

Vestibular dysfunction in Long COVID often coexists with other neurological or autonomic issues, complicating treatment and prognosis. More research is needed to understand the long-term outcomes and best practices for managing these symptoms.

Understanding the connection between the vestibular system and Long COVID provides insight into why some patients continue to experience disabling symptoms long after the acute phase of the illness has passed.

Symptom Summary by Cause

Any of the symptoms are common between Long COVID, ME/CFS, and POTS. This list describes which cause can create what symptoms. This summary helps you determine which causes are the most prominent. It is essential because you can sometimes have more than one cause. That's ok. They are all connected. Treat the most prominent one first.

Symptom	Dysautonomia	Mitochondrial dysfunction	Gut Dysbiosis	Histamine /MCAS
Abdominal bloating	x	x	xx	x
Abdominal pain	x	x	x	x
Abnormal smell or taste/anosmia/ parosmia/ dysgeusia	x			
Acid Reflux / GERD	x		x	x
Anxiety	xx		x	x
Bladder control issues	x			x
Blurry vision/ double vision	x	x		
Body pains	x	x		x
Brain fog/loss of executive functions	x	x	x	x
Burning mouth	x		x	

Changes in voice	xx[2]		x	
Chest pain/tightness	x	x		x
Coat hanger pain (head, neck, shoulders)	x			
Concentration problems	x			
Cough	x			x
Depression/ derealization/depersonalization	x		x	
Diarrhea	x	x	x	x
Symptom	**Dysautonomia**	**Mitochondrial dysfunction**	**Gut Dysbiosis**	**Histamine /MCAS**
Dizziness	x			
Dry eyes	x			
Exercise intolerance	x	xx		
Fatigue	x	x	x	
Fever	x			
Gastroparesis	x	x	x	
Hair loss	x			
Headache/head pressure	x			x
Increased light, sound, and smell sensitivity (sensory overload)	x			
Insomnia / don't feel refreshed after waking	x		x	x
Insulin resistance		x	x	
Irritability	x			

Joint pain (arthralgia)	x		x	
Memory problems	x			
Menstrual cycle /period changes/change in libido / sexual dysfunction	x		x	x
Mitochondrial dysfunction		X	1	
Muscle aches (myalgia)	x	x		
Muscle fasciculations	x	xx		
Muscle weakness		xx		
Nausea	x	x	xx	x
Neuropathies/ vibrations/pins and needles (1)	x	x	x [1]	
Post-Exertional Malaise (PEM)	x	xx		
POTS	x	x		
PTSD	x			
Rashes	x			
Symptom	**Dysautonomia**	**Mitochondrial dysfunction**	**Gut Dysbiosis**	**Histamine /MCAS**
Shortness of breath	x	xx		x
Sore throat	x			
Stuffy nose, post nasal drip	x			x
Tachycardia	x			x
Temperature intolerance / hot flashes /	x			

inappropriate sweating				
Tinnitus	xx			
Tremors/ twitching	x			
Trouble swallowing / lump in the throat	xx	x		
Vertigo	x			
Vitamin deficiency			x	
Weight gain/loss	x	x	x	

- Thru malabsorption of B vitamins [1]
- Vagus nerve dysfunction [2]

Dysautonomia Symptoms

Cardiovascular Symptoms

- **Dizziness and Lightheadedness:** You might feel dizzy or lightheaded, especially when you stand up quickly. This happens because your blood pressure drops suddenly (a condition called orthostatic hypotension).

- **Fainting (Syncope):** Some people experience fainting spells or near-fainting episodes, also related to blood pressure drops and inadequate blood flow to the brain.

- **Rapid Heart Rate (Tachycardia):** Your heart might race or pound, even when you're resting. This is common in a form of dysautonomia called Postural Orthostatic Tachycardia Syndrome (POTS).

- **Chest Pain:** You might feel chest discomfort or pain, which can be concerning but is often due to changes in heart rate and blood pressure. It is important to still rule out heart and lung related issues such as myocarditis, pericarditis, angina, and lung related problems.

Gastrointestinal Symptoms

- **Nausea:** You might feel nauseous frequently, as if you have an upset stomach.
- **Bloating and Abdominal Pain:** Your stomach might feel full and bloated, and you might have cramps or pain.
- **Constipation or Diarrhea:** You might experience difficulty having regular bowel movements (constipation) or have frequent, loose stools (diarrhea).
- **Difficulty Swallowing (Dysphagia):** It might be hard to swallow food or drinks, which can lead to choking or a feeling of food being stuck.

Neurological Symptoms

- **Headaches and Migraines:** Frequent headaches or migraines can be a symptom, often due to changes in blood flow or pressure in the brain.
- **Brain Fog:** You might have trouble concentrating, remembering things, or thinking clearly. It can feel like a mental cloudiness or confusion.
- **Fatigue:** Feeling extremely tired all the time, even after a good night's sleep, is very common. This fatigue can be overwhelming and debilitating.
- **Swallowing problems**
- **Voice change, hoarse voice**
- **Coat hanger pain**
- **Tinnitus**
- **Tingling and Numbness (neuropathies)**

  - You might feel pins and needles, tingling, or numbness in your hands and feet, which is related to nerve issues.
  - These can show up as internal vibrations and can affect any area of the body.

Respiratory Symptoms

- **Shortness of Breath:** You might feel like you can't catch your breath or are breathing more quickly than usual, even with minimal exertion.

Temperature Regulation Issues

- **Sweating Too Much or Too Little:** You might sweat excessively, even in cool temperatures, or not at all, even when it's hot. Both are signs that your body can't regulate temperature properly.
- **Feeling Hot or Cold:** You might feel too hot or too cold without a clear reason, as your body struggles to maintain a normal temperature.
- **Cold hands or cold feet**

Urinary Symptoms

- **Frequent Urination:** You might need to urinate more often than usual.
- **Difficulty Urinating:** You might find it hard to start urinating or feel like your bladder isn't emptying completely.

Sleep Problems

- **Insomnia:** Difficulty falling or staying asleep is common. You might wake up frequently during the night or have restless, unrefreshing sleep. Even if you get the 7-8 hours of sleep a night or longer, if you still feel tired, it's still not a good quality sleep.

- **Sleep Apnea:** This is a condition where your breathing stops and starts during sleep usually due to an airway obstruction. Snoring is common. It can leave you feeling tired even after a full night's sleep.

Musculoskeletal Symptoms

- **Muscle Weakness and Pain:** You might experience weakness in your muscles, making it hard to perform everyday tasks. Muscle pain (also known as myalgia) and aches can also be present.

- **Joint Pain:** Joint pain (also known as arthralgia) and discomfort are also common and can be mistaken for other conditions like arthritis.

Psychological Symptoms

Anxiety and Depression: Chronic illness can lead to feelings of anxiety and depression. The unpredictability of symptoms and their impact on daily life can be stressful and emotionally challenging.

- Anxiety
- Depression
- PTSD
- Derealization
- Depersonalization

Sensory Symptoms

Light and Sound Senses Changes

You might become overly sensitive to bright lights and loud noises, which can trigger headaches or discomfort. Unlike previously thought, the changes in smell and taste are not due to brain damage. There are subtle changes in blood flow and the chronic inflammatory environment surrounding the olfactory neurons that may be responsible. It is often instantly corrected after a stellate ganglion block, suggesting a different mechanism at work.

About 70-90% of what we consider taste actually comes from smell. You may have noticed that taste is muted during a cold, flu, or sinus infection. That is due to inflammation of the olfactory system rather than taste buds.

Taste and smell abnormality

- **Anosmia** – absence of smell
- **Ageusia** – absence of taste
- **Parosmia** – abnormal smells (pleasant or unpleasant)
- **Dysgeusia** – abnormal taste (pleasant or unpleasant)
- **Phantosmia** (olfactory hallucination) – sensing smells that are not there
- Increased sensitivity to taste and smell

Tinnitus

- commonly described as a ringing, buzzing, or hissing sound in the ears, has been reported as a symptom experienced by some individuals with Long COVID. Here's an explanation of tinnitus in the context of Long COVID, including potential causes, mechanisms, and implications:

General Symptoms

- **Exercise Intolerance:** Physical activity might make you feel worse, causing extreme fatigue or dizziness. This makes it hard to stay active and fit.

- **Post Exertional Malaise (PEM):** Imagine your body is like a car. Normally, when you use energy to do things like walk, study, or play, your body can "refuel" and get back to normal quickly, just like a car needs gasoline to keep going. For people with PEM, their bodies don't refuel properly. Instead, after doing something active, they feel really tired, sick, and it can take a long time to recover – much longer than it does for most people. These symptoms can appear right after doing an activity or a day or two later, and they can last for days, weeks, or even longer. The autonomic nervous system, which controls things like heart rate and blood pressure, might be out of balance in people with PEM, leading to their symptoms.

Mitochondrial Dysfunction Symptoms

General Symptoms

- **Fatigue:** Persistent, unexplained tiredness that is not relieved by rest.
- **Exercise Intolerance:** Difficulty in performing physical activities, leading to rapid exhaustion and muscle weakness.

Neurological Symptoms

- **Muscle Weakness:** Especially noticeable in muscles that require high energy, such as those in the limbs.
- **Neuropathy:** Numbness, tingling, or pain in the extremities due to nerve damage.
- **Seizures:** Episodes of uncontrolled electrical activity in the brain.
- **Developmental Delays:** In children, delayed milestones in motor skills, speech, and cognitive development.
- **Movement Disorders:** Tremors, spasms, or involuntary movements.
- **Ataxia:** Loss of coordination and balance, leading to clumsiness or unsteady gait.

- **Cognitive Impairment:** Difficulties with memory, concentration, and other cognitive functions.

Gastrointestinal Symptoms

- **Feeding Difficulties:** Problems with swallowing or digesting food.

- **Constipation or Diarrhea:** Irregular bowel movements due to impaired gastrointestinal motility.

- **Vomiting and Nausea:** Frequent episodes, often associated with energy metabolism issues in the gastrointestinal tract.

- **Gastroparesis:** Delayed stomach emptying, leading to bloating, discomfort, and malnutrition.

Cardiovascular Symptoms

- **Cardiomyopathy:** Disease of the heart muscle, leading to weakened heart function and heart failure.

- **Arrhythmias:** Irregular heartbeats that can be too fast, too slow, or erratic.

- **Hypotension:** Low blood pressure, especially upon standing (orthostatic hypotension).

Respiratory Symptoms

- **Breathing Difficulties:** Shortness of breath, especially during physical exertion.

- **Respiratory Muscle Weakness:** Leading to ineffective breathing and potential respiratory failure.

Endocrine Symptoms

- **Diabetes Mellitus**: Particularly insulin resistance and type 2 diabetes.

- **Thyroid Dysfunction:** Hypothyroidism or hyperthyroidism due to impaired energy metabolism in the thyroid gland.

Visual and Auditory Symptoms

- **Vision Problems:** Progressive external ophthalmoplegia (weakness of the eye muscles), optic neuropathy, or retinopathy. This can result in double vision and blurry vision.

- **Hearing Loss:** Sensorineural hearing loss, often progressive.

Renal Symptoms

- **Kidney Dysfunction:** Impaired ability to filter waste, leading to conditions like Fanconi syndrome, characterized by excess loss of nutrients in urine.

Hematological Symptoms

- **Anemia:** Low red blood cell count, leading to fatigue and pallor.

- **Lactic Acidosis:** Buildup of lactic acid in the blood, leading to muscle cramps, nausea, and rapid breathing.

Dermatological Symptoms

- **Skin Rashes:** Various types of skin conditions may occur.

- **Hair Loss:** Thinning or loss of hair due to poor energy production affecting hair follicles.

Musculoskeletal Symptoms

- **Myopathy:** Muscle pain and cramping, especially after exercise.

- **Osteopenia/Osteoporosis:** Decreased bone density, leading to brittle bones and fractures.

- **Mitochondrial Myopathy:** Muscle weakness, exercise intolerance, and cramps.

- **Exercise Intolerance:** Physical activity might make you feel worse, causing extreme fatigue or dizziness. This makes it hard to stay active and fit.

Gut Dysbiosis Symptoms

An imbalance in the gut microbiota, affects not only the gastrointestinal system but also various other bodily functions due to the gut's connection to the immune, metabolic, and nervous systems. Here are **non-gastrointestinal symptoms** associated with gut dysbiosis:

1. Neurological and Cognitive Symptoms

- **Brain Fog**: Difficulty concentrating, memory issues, or mental fatigue is common, often due to the gut-brain axis and the influence of gut bacteria on cognitive function.

- **Mood Disorders**: Dysbiosis can affect mental health, leading to **anxiety**, **depression**, or increased irritability. Gut bacteria produce neurotransmitters like serotonin, so an imbalance can lead to mood swings or emotional instability.

- **Headaches and Migraines**: Certain bacterial imbalances may trigger headaches or migraines through inflammatory processes and changes in gut permeability.

- **Sleep Disturbances**: Gut dysbiosis may lead to insomnia or poor sleep quality, often linked to disrupted serotonin and melatonin production.

2. Immune System-Related Symptoms

- **Frequent Infections**: A weakened immune response due to dysbiosis can make you more susceptible to infections, including colds, flu, or sinus infections.

- **Chronic Inflammation**: Dysbiosis can trigger systemic inflammation, which may manifest as body aches, joint pain, or a general feeling of unwellness.
- **Autoimmune Disorders**: An imbalanced gut can contribute to the development or worsening of autoimmune diseases, such as **rheumatoid arthritis**, **Hashimoto's thyroiditis**, or **lupus**, through immune dysregulation.
- **Allergic Reactions**: Increased food sensitivities, histamine intolerance, or skin conditions like eczema can be related to immune system disruptions from gut dysbiosis.

3. Skin Conditions

- **Acne**: Dysbiosis is associated with skin problems like acne, often related to inflammation and toxin buildup from poor gut health.
- **Eczema**: Imbalances in gut bacteria can exacerbate eczema or other dermatitis conditions, potentially due to immune system dysregulation.
- **Rosacea**: Gut dysbiosis has been linked to rosacea, possibly through inflammation and immune responses triggered by gut-related toxins.

4. Metabolic Symptoms

- **Weight Gain or Obesity**: Imbalances in the gut microbiota can affect metabolism and promote fat storage, leading to weight gain or difficulty losing weight.
- **Insulin Resistance**: Dysbiosis may contribute to metabolic syndrome and insulin resistance, which can lead to type 2 diabetes.
- **Blood Sugar Dysregulation**: Some people may experience frequent blood sugar spikes or drops, contributing to symptoms like fatigue, dizziness, and sugar cravings.

5. Chronic Fatigue

- **Energy Imbalance**: Dysbiosis can reduce the absorption of nutrients, leading to chronic fatigue. It also affects the production of certain vitamins (e.g., B vitamins) and neurotransmitters necessary for energy metabolism.

- **Mitochondrial Dysfunction**: A disrupted gut microbiome can affect mitochondrial function, further contributing to fatigue and weakness.

6. Respiratory Symptoms

- **Asthma and Allergic Rhinitis**: Dysbiosis is linked to increased susceptibility to respiratory conditions like asthma, due to immune dysregulation and increased inflammation.

- **Non-Allergic Rhinitis**: Gut dysbiosis may play a role in the inflammation of nasal passages, leading to non-allergic nasal congestion or runny nose.

7. Cardiovascular Symptoms

- **High Blood Pressure**: Certain bacterial imbalances may promote inflammation that contributes to hypertension or other cardiovascular issues.

- **Cholesterol Imbalances**: Dysbiosis can affect lipid metabolism, potentially leading to elevated cholesterol levels and an increased risk of cardiovascular diseases.

8. Musculoskeletal Symptoms

- **Joint Pain**: Dysbiosis-related inflammation can lead to joint and muscle pain, particularly in conditions like rheumatoid arthritis or fibromyalgia.

- **Muscle Weakness**: Chronic inflammation and poor nutrient absorption due to gut dysbiosis can contribute to muscle weakness or cramps.

9. Hormonal Imbalances

- **Thyroid Dysfunction**: Dysbiosis can lead to immune-related thyroid conditions (e.g., Hashimoto's thyroiditis) and hormonal imbalances, affecting metabolism and energy levels.

- **Estrogen Imbalance**: The gut is involved in the regulation of estrogen levels. Dysbiosis can lead to excess estrogen (estrogen dominance), which can contribute to conditions like **PMS**, **fibroids**, or **endometriosis**.

- **Menstrual Irregularities**: Hormonal imbalances linked to gut dysbiosis can cause irregular or painful menstrual cycles and worsen symptoms of **PMS** or **PMDD** (premenstrual dysphoric disorder).

10. Food Intolerances and Sensitivities

- **Increased Sensitivity to Foods**: Dysbiosis can lead to non-allergic food sensitivities, including reactions to gluten, dairy, or other common triggers, as gut permeability and immune regulation are affected.

- **Histamine Intolerance**: Dysbiosis can lead to poor histamine breakdown, leading to histamine-related symptoms such as headaches, flushing, and nasal congestion.

11. Poor Nutrient Absorption

- **Vitamin Deficiencies**: Gut dysbiosis can impair the absorption of key vitamins and minerals, leading to deficiencies, particularly in **vitamin B12**, **vitamin D**, **magnesium**, and **iron**, contributing to symptoms like anemia, fatigue, or poor immune function.

Excess Histamine

Beyond allergic reactions, histamine can cause a variety of symptoms throughout the body due to its role in immune response, neurotransmission, and regulation of physiological functions. Because the other symptoms tend to mimic the other causes, it is useful to look for runny nose, itchy eyes, hives and other allergy related histamine symptoms to see if histamine is involved.

Non-allergic symptoms related to high histamine levels, often referred to as **histamine intolerance** or dysregulation:

1. Gastrointestinal Symptoms

- **Diarrhea**: Histamine promotes gastric acid secretion and motility, which can lead to diarrhea, especially after eating histamine-rich foods.
- **Bloating**: High histamine levels can lead to increased gas production and bloating.
- **Abdominal Pain**: Histamine can trigger intestinal cramping and discomfort.
- **Nausea and Vomiting**: These can occur due to histamine's effect on the gut and its involvement in the brain's vomiting center.

2. Cardiovascular Symptoms

- **Low Blood Pressure (Hypotension)**: Histamine causes blood vessel dilation, which can lead to a drop in blood pressure.
- **Heart Palpitations or Tachycardia**: Increased histamine levels can stimulate heart rate and cause irregular or rapid heartbeats.
- **Dizziness or Lightheadedness**: Due to vasodilation and hypotension, high histamine can lead to dizziness or fainting.

3. Neurological Symptoms

- **Headaches and Migraines**: Histamine acts as a neurotransmitter and can trigger headaches, particularly migraines, due to blood vessel dilation and neuroinflammation.
- **Brain Fog**: Difficulty concentrating or cognitive impairment is often associated with high histamine levels.
- **Anxiety or Irritability**: Histamine is involved in regulating mood and anxiety levels through its action in the central nervous system.
    - **Histamine and Anxiety Disorders:** Elevated levels of histamine have been observed in patients **with panic disorder** and **generalized anxiety disorder (GAD)**.
- **Insomnia**: Histamine acts as a wakefulness-promoting agent in the brain, so elevated levels can interfere with sleep, leading to difficulty falling or staying asleep.
- **Tingling or Numbness**: Neurological symptoms like tingling sensations or numbness in the extremities may be linked to histamine dysregulation.

4. Respiratory Symptoms (Non-Allergic)

- **Nasal Congestion or Runny Nose (Non-Allergic Rhinitis)**: Even without allergies, histamine can cause chronic nasal congestion, runny nose, or postnasal drip.
- **Difficulty Breathing or Shortness of Breath**: Histamine constricts the smooth muscles in the bronchi, which may lead to breathing difficulties.

5. Skin Symptoms

- **Flushing or Redness**: Excess histamine can cause the blood vessels in the skin to dilate, leading to facial flushing or redness.

- **Hives or Urticaria** (Non-Allergic): Histamine can trigger itchy, raised welts (hives), even without an allergic trigger.

- **Sweating**: Histamine can induce sweating, particularly after consuming histamine-rich foods.

6. Reproductive System Symptoms

- **Menstrual Irregularities**: High histamine levels can interfere with hormone balance and may lead to menstrual cycle irregularities, including painful periods (dysmenorrhea).

- **Premenstrual Syndrome (PMS)**: Elevated histamine is linked to worsening PMS symptoms, including mood swings and bloating.

7. Urinary and Genitourinary Symptoms

- **Frequent Urination**: Histamine can act on the bladder, leading to more frequent urination, particularly at night (nocturia).

- **Interstitial Cystitis**: Histamine is thought to contribute to bladder inflammation and pain, characteristic of interstitial cystitis (painful bladder syndrome).

8. Joint and Muscle Symptoms

- **Muscle Pain or Cramps**: High histamine levels can lead to muscle aches or cramps, possibly due to its effect on smooth muscles or inflammation.

- **Joint Pain**: Histamine can promote inflammation in joints, leading to stiffness or pain, especially in conditions like histamine intolerance.

9. Eye Symptoms

- **Non-Allergic Conjunctivitis**: Histamine can cause watery, irritated, or red eyes even in the absence of an allergic trigger.

10. General Symptoms

- **Fatigue**: Histamine imbalance can cause chronic fatigue or a feeling of being "run-down."
- **Food Sensitivities**: People with histamine intolerance may react to foods high in histamine (e.g., aged cheese, fermented foods, alcohol), experiencing gastrointestinal, neurological, or cardiovascular symptoms.

References:

1. Xu, E., Xie, Y. & Al-Aly, Z. Long-term gastrointestinal outcomes of COVID-19. *Nat Commun* **14**, 983 (2023). https://doi.org/10.1038/s41467-023-36223-7
2. Davis HE, McCorkell L, Vogel JM, Topol EJ. Long COVID: major findings, mechanisms and recommendations. Nat Rev Microbiol. 2023 Mar;21(3):133-146. doi: 10.1038/s41579-022-00846-2. Epub 2023 Jan 13. Erratum in: Nat Rev Microbiol. 2023 Jun;21(6):408. doi: 10.1038/s41579-023-00896-0. PMID: 36639608; PMCID: PMC9839201.
3. Burges Watson DL, Campbell M, Hopkins C, Smith B, Kelly C, Deary V. Altered smell and taste: Anosmia, parosmia and the impact of long Covid-19. PLoS One. 2021 Sep 24;16(9):e0256998. doi: 10.1371/journal.pone.0256998. PMID: 34559820; PMCID: PMC8462678.
4. Sequeira Rodriguez, P., Santana Ortiz, R., & Ortiz-Hernández, E. (2023). Late onset and persistent parosmia and dysgeusia as neurosensorial complication by the SARS virus COV 2. *Otolaryngology Case Reports, 26*, 100510. https://doi.org/10.1016/j.xocr.2023.100510
5. Rogn, Å., Jensen, J.L., Iversen, P.O. *et al.* Publisher Correction: Post-COVID-19 patients suffer from chemosensory, trigeminal, and salivary dysfunctions. *Sci Rep* **14**, 9213 (2024). https://doi.org/10.1038/s41598-024-59915-6

6. Tan, B. K. J., Han, R., Zhao, J. J., Tan, N. K. W., Quah, E. S. H., & Tan, C. J.-W. (2022). Prognosis and persistence of smell and taste dysfunction in patients with COVID-19: Meta-analysis with parametric cure modelling of recovery curves. *BMJ*, 378, e069503. https://doi.org/10.1136/bmj-2021-069503

7. Davis, H.E., McCorkell, L., Vogel, J.M. *et al.* Long COVID: major findings, mechanisms and recommendations. *Nat Rev Microbiol* **21**, 133–146 (2023). https://doi.org/10.1038/s41579-022-00846-2

8. Ebner, B., Volz, Y., Mumm, JN. *et al.* The COVID-19 pandemic — what have urologists learned? *Nat Rev Urol* **19**, 344–356 (2022). https://doi.org/10.1038/s41585-022-00586-1

9. Aubin MS, Shridharani A, Barboi AC, Guralnick ML, Jaradeh SS, Prieto TE, O'Connor RC. Lower urinary tract dysfunction in patients with dysautonomia. Clin Auton Res. 2015 Dec;25(6):407-10. doi: 10.1007/s10286-015-0320-z. Epub 2015 Nov 3. PMID: 26530163.

10. Jones, B. M., & Tykocki, N. R. (2020). New direct evidence that histamine augments bladder sensory outflow during filling is nothing to sneeze at. *American Journal of Physiology-Renal Physiology*, *318*(2), F455–F456.

11. Hejbøl, E. K., Harbo, T., Agergaard, J., Madsen, L. B., Pedersen, T. H., Østergaard, L. J., Andersen, H., Schrøder, H. D., & Tankisi, H. (2022). Myopathy as a cause of fatigue in long-term post-COVID-19 symptoms: Evidence of skeletal muscle histopathology. *European Journal of Neurology*. Advance online publication. https://doi.org/10.1111/ene.15435

12. Chen TH, Chang CJ, Hung PH. Possible Pathogenesis and Prevention of Long COVID: SARS-CoV-2-Induced Mitochondrial Disorder. Int J Mol Sci. 2023 Apr 28;24(9):8034. doi: 10.3390/ijms24098034. PMID: 37175745; PMCID: PMC10179190.

13. Pollack, B., von Saltza, E., McCorkell, L., Santos, L., Hultman, A., Cohen, A. K., & Soares, L. (2023). Female reproductive health

impacts of Long COVID and associated illnesses including ME/CFS, POTS, and connective tissue disorders: A literature review. *Frontiers in Rehabilitation Science*, 4, Article 1122673. https://doi.org/10.3389/fresc.2023.1122673

14. Moura das Neves, P. F., Quaresma, J. A. S., Queiroz, M. A. F., Silva, C. C., Maia, E. V., de Sousa Oliveira, J. S., Almeida das Neves, C. M., Mendonça, S. S., Falcão, A. S. C., Melo, G. S., Santos, I. B. F., de Sousa, J. R., dos Santos, E. J. M., da Costa Vasconcelos, P. F., Vallinoto, A. C. R., & Falcão, L. F. M. (2023). Imbalance of peripheral temperature, sympathovagal, and cytokine profile in Long COVID. *Biology (Basel)*, 12(5), Article 749. https://doi.org/10.3390/biology12050749

15. Buoite Stella, A., Furlanis, G., Frezza, N.A. *et al.* Autonomic dysfunction in post-COVID patients with and without neurological symptoms: a prospective multidomain observational study. *J Neurol* **269**, 587–596 (2022). https://doi.org/10.1007/s00415-021-10735-y

16. Zhang, D., Zhou, Y., Ma, Y., Chen, P., Tang, J., Yang, B., Li, H., Liang, M., Xue, Y., Liu, Y., Zhang, J., & Wang, X. (2023). Gut microbiota dysbiosis correlates with Long COVID-19 at one year after discharge. *Journal of Korean Medical Science*, 38(15), Article e120. https://doi.org/10.3346/jkms.2023.38.e120

17. Raciti L, De Luca R, Raciti G, Arcadi FA, Calabrò RS. The Use of Palmitoylethanolamide in the Treatment of Long COVID: A Real-Life Retrospective Cohort Study. Med Sci (Basel). 2022 Jul 14;10(3):37. doi: 10.3390/medsci10030037. PMID: 35893119; PMCID: PMC9326613.

Autoimmunity in Long COVID

Dysautonomia, a disorder of the Autonomic Nervous System (ANS), can contribute to immune dysregulation and potentially lead to autoimmunity. When discussing autoimmune conditions, we sometimes observe in Long COVID, these are similar but not exactly like their counterparts, such as diabetes, rheumatoid arthritis, lupus (SLE), Sjogren's syndrome, and thyroiditis. Typically, the Antinuclear Antibody **(ANA) blood test** will be elevated, but nothing else.

How Dysautonomia Leads to Immune Dysregulation

The ANS is integral in modulating the immune system. Dysregulation of the ANS can impact immune function through several mechanisms:

1. **Stress Response:** Dysautonomia can lead to an altered stress response involving excessive or insufficient release of stress hormones like cortisol. Chronic stress and abnormal cortisol levels can suppress or dysregulate immune function.

2. **Inflammatory Pathways:** The ANS influences the release of cytokines (big ones are IL-1, IL-6, TNF-α), which are critical mediators of inflammation. Dysautonomia can disrupt this balance, leading to excessive inflammation or an inadequate immune response.

3. **Blood Flow and Organ Function:** Impaired blood flow due to dysautonomia can impact the function of immune organs such as the spleen and lymph nodes, leading to compromised immune surveillance and response.

Dysautonomia and Autoimmunity

Dysautonomia might contribute in multiple ways to the development of autoimmunity:

1. **Molecular Mimicry:** Dysautonomia can arise following infections that also trigger autoimmunity. For instance, a viral infection might cause an immune response that inadvertently targets the body's own tissues (molecular mimicry), including those of the ANS.

2. **Chronic Inflammation:** Persistent dysregulation of the ANS can lead to chronic inflammation, creating an environment that promotes the development of autoimmunity. Chronic inflammation can cause continuous immune system activation, increasing the risk of autoimmunity.

3. **Altered Immune Regulation:** Dysautonomia can disrupt the typical regulatory mechanisms of the immune system, such as the function of regulatory T cells, which help inhibit autoimmunity. Impaired regulation can lead to an increased likelihood of autoimmune responses.

Long COVID, Dysautonomia, and Autoimmunity

In the context of Long COVID, many patients report symptoms consistent with dysautonomia, such as POTS. The SARS-CoV-2 virus can cause damage to the autonomic nervous system, either directly through viral invasion or indirectly through inflammation and immune-mediated damage.

1. **Post-Infectious Dysautonomia:** Viral infections—including COVID-19—can lead to dysautonomia as a post-infectious complication. It can result from direct damage to autonomic nerves or immune responses triggered by the infection.

2. **Chronic Inflammation and Autoimmunity:** Persistent autonomic dysfunction can maintain a state of chronic inflammation, which might contribute to developing or exacerbating autoimmune conditions. The

ongoing immune activation in dysautonomia can increase the risk of autoimmunity in vulnerable individuals.

Autoimmune Conditions Associated with Long COVID?

Neurological Autoimmune Conditions

1. **Guillain-Barré Syndrome (GBS)**
2. **Multiple Sclerosis (MS) Exacerbation**
3. **Autoimmune Encephalitis**
4. **Myasthenia Gravis (MG)**
5. **Small Fiber Neuropathy (SFN)**
6. **Neuromyelitis Optica Spectrum Disorder (NMOSD)**
7. **Autoimmune Dysautonomia** (including Postural Orthostatic Tachycardia Syndrome - POTS).

Rheumatologic and Musculoskeletal Autoimmune Conditions

1. **Rheumatoid Arthritis (RA)**: both new onset and flares of existing disease.
2. **Systemic Lupus Erythematosus (SLE)**: both new onset and flares of existing disease.
3. **Polymyalgia Rheumatica (PMR)**: This inflammatory disorder causing muscle pain and stiffness, primarily in the shoulders and hips.
4. **Inflammatory Myopathies**: Conditions like dermatomyositis and polymyositis, which cause muscle inflammation and weakness,

Endocrine Autoimmune Conditions

1. **Autoimmune Thyroiditis** (e.g., Hashimoto's thyroiditis, Graves' disease): Thyroid dysfunction has been reported, with some cases of autoimmune thyroiditis triggered or exacerbated.

2. **Type 1 Diabetes Mellitus**: New-onset type 1 diabetes has been observed in some Long COVID patients, potentially due to autoimmune attack on pancreatic beta cells.

Gastrointestinal Autoimmune Conditions

1. **Celiac Disease**: trigger or exacerbate celiac disease.

2. **Autoimmune Hepatitis**: Liver inflammation due to an autoimmune response has been reported in some Long COVID patients.

3. **Inflammatory Bowel Disease (IBD)**: Flares in Crohn's disease and ulcerative colitis have been noted.

Dermatologic Autoimmune Conditions

1. **Psoriasis**: new-onset psoriasis or worsening of existing psoriasis.

2. **Lichen Planus**: An inflammatory condition that affects the skin and mucous membranes.

3. **Vitiligo**: Reports have suggested that COVID-19 might trigger or worsen vitiligo, a condition where the immune system attacks melanocytes, leading to depigmented skin patches.

Hematologic Autoimmune Conditions

1. **Autoimmune Hemolytic Anemia (AIHA)**: A condition where the immune system attacks red blood cells, leading to anemia.

2. **Immune Thrombocytopenic Purpura (ITP)**: ITP, where the immune system attacks platelets, causing low platelet counts.

3. **Antiphospholipid Syndrome (APS)**

    - COVID-19 has been linked to the development of antiphospholipid antibodies, which can lead to APS, a condition that increases the risk of blood clots.

Cardiovascular Autoimmune Conditions

1. **Myocarditis and Pericarditis**
    - These inflammatory conditions of the heart muscle and surrounding tissue, often autoimmune in nature, have been linked to COVID-19.
2. **Kawasaki-like Syndrome** or Multisystem Inflammatory Syndrome in Children (**MIS-C**)
    - A severe inflammatory syndrome in children resembling Kawasaki disease, which can cause coronary artery aneurysms, has been associated with COVID-19.

Miscellaneous Autoimmune Conditions

1. **Sjögren's Syndrome**
    - COVID-19 has been reported to trigger or worsen Sjögren's syndrome, which affects the glands that produce moisture.
2. **Sarcoidosis**
    - An inflammatory disease that can affect multiple organs, especially the lungs and lymph glands, potentially linked to COVID-19.
3. **Vasculitis**
    - Inflammation of blood vessels, including conditions like giant cell arteritis and ANCA-associated vasculitis, has been reported post-COVID-19.

References:

1. Sharma, C., Bayry, J. High risk of autoimmune diseases after COVID-19. *Nat Rev Rheumatol* **19**, 399–400 (2023).

   https://DOI.org/10.1038/s41584-023-00964-y

2. Son K, Jamil R, Chowdhury A, Mukherjee M, Venegas C, Miyasaki K, Zhang K, Patel Z, Salter B, Yuen ACY, Lau KSK, Cowbrough B, Radford K, Huang C, Kjarsgaard M, Dvorkin-Gheva A, Smith J, Li QZ, Waserman S, Ryerson CJ, Nair P, Ho T, Balakrishnan N, Nazy I, Bowdish DME, Svenningsen S, Carlsten C, Mukherjee M. Circulating anti-nuclear autoantibodies in COVID-19 survivors predict Long COVID symptoms. *Eur Respir J*. 2023;61(1):2200970.

   DOI:10.1183/13993003.00970-2022.

Initial Labs for Diagnosis

I know people want answers. Do I really have Long COVID? What is wrong with me? These labs are not meant to diagnose Long COVID. Labs and urine analysis are essential to determine if any other conditions are contributing to Long COVID and if there are any dangerous conditions, such as pericarditis, myocarditis, kidney stones, liver problems, and kidney problems, may need to be addressed first before treating Long COVID. Sure, you can order a massive catalog of tests and spend thousands. At the end of the day, though, most will not enlighten you on what is wrong. These tests will not diagnose if you have Long COVID as there is no test or diagnostic to do that. However, we can get clues to the causes of the Long COVID by looking for mitochondrial dysfunction and histamine involvement in addition to the symptoms. It is often unnecessary to do extensive autoimmune and cytokine panels or expensive genetic testing because the results will not change the treatments.

> *"I have had patients bring in literal books of labs—hundreds of pages. I do review them, but I have found that I only look at a few, the ones that will change what I will do. The majority of the labs are not useful to me. Remember, medicine is as much an art as a science. It has to make sense to me."*

Blood work

1. **CBC** with differential and platelet count

2. Standard blood chemistries (**Basic Metabolic Profile (BMP) or blood chemistry panel**)
3. liver function tests (AST, ALT, bilirubin)
4. kidney/renal function tests
5. **D-Dimer**—as a marker of clotting activation.
6. **Fibrinogen level**
7. **Thrombin generation assays (TGA)** and specific markers of thrombin formation. Like elevated **Factor XIIa** or **prekallikrein activation.**
8. **C- Reactive Protein (CRP)** —a marker of ongoing inflammation. A comprehensive, extensive cytokine/chemokine panel is unnecessary and extremely expensive, and the results will not change the treatment approach.
9. **Early morning cortisol**—some patients develop autoimmune adrenal failure. It also helps diagnose Long COVID. Cortisol can be tracked throughout the day as well.
10. **TSH, free T3, T4**—to exclude thyroid disease
11. **Homocysteine level** – an amino acid that encourages blood clotting. Vascular damage marker
12. **HbA1C**—Vaccine-injured and Long COVID patients are at an increased risk of developing diabetes
13. **Troponin** and **pro-BNP** to exclude cardiac disease.
14. **Vitamin D** level (25-OH Vitamin D)
15. **Vitamin levels B1, B2, B3, B5, B6, B9, B12**
16. **Ferritin** – iron deficiency marker
17. **Serotonin level**
18. **Optional to check for reactivation**
    a. Cytomegalovirus (CMV)

b. Ebstein Barr Virus (EBV) - early antigen IgG or nuclear antigen IgG

c. Herpes simplex

d. exanthem/sixth disease/roseola (HHV-6, 7 or 8)

e. mycoplasma serology/PCR

f. Lyme disease (chronic Lyme disease is controversial), but undiagnosed and untreated Lyme is genuine.

g. Bartonella (passed by fleas, ticks, and other vectors)

h. Babesia tick-borne diseases

19. **Optional for MCAS**

a. Serum tryptase (tends to only be elevated if tested within 2-3 hours of *anaphylaxis*)

b. serum histamine

c. 24-h urine N-methylhistamine

20. **Optional autoimmune**

a. Lupus anticoagulant and ANA

21. **Optional for Mitochondria dysfunction:**

a. pyruvate/lactate

b. mitochondrial DNA number

Summary of Treatment Options for Each Cause

Most available treatment options are summarized in the following table. However, it does not imply you should take all of them simultaneously (as in, don't take all of them at the same time). The selection of supplements and medications requires clinical and medical judgment.

Cause and mechanisms	Treatment ideas/possibilities
Dysautonomia – can occur from damage to the vagus nerve, low serotonin,	The goal here is to: • Symptomatically treat POTS • rebalance the autonomic nervous system by improving vagus nerve function and reducing fight or flight. Pyridostigmine, Huperzine A, *Stellate Ganglion Block* (SGB), VNS, Epipharyngeal Abrasive Therapy (EAT), nicotine patch (14 days or less) POTS only: fludrocortisone, beta-blockers, corlinor (ivabradine), Midodrine
Mitochondrial dysfunction – can develop due to direct viral damage to mitochondrial DNA, electron chain disruption, accumulation of abnormal proteins inside mitochondria, or	The goal here is to: • Remove damaged mitochondria (mitophagy) • Eliminate damaged cells (autophagy) • Increase mitochondria numbers in healthy cells • Improve mitochondrial function by making it easier for them to perform their job • Support mitochondrial metabolic mechanisms

malabsorption of critical vitamins.	• Reduce oxidative stress Antioxidants, intermittent fasting, pacing, respiratory rehab, physical therapy, apigenin, Citrulline/arginine, d-ribose, membrane phospholipids, Palmitoylethanolamide (PEA), CoQ10, NAD+/NMN/NR, L-carnitine, alpha-ketoglutaric acid, honokiol, dichloroacetate, alpha lipoid acid (ALA), magnesium, calcium, phosphate, vitamin B1, B2, B3, B5, B9, B12, creatine, calcium pyruvate, PQQ, urolithin A, rapamycin, metformin, MOTS-C, SS-31 The ones listed below can minimize oxidative stress from their antioxidant effects. **Antioxidants:** Quercetin, curcumin, rutin, fisetin, hesperidin, kaempferol, apigenin, luteolin, molecular hydrogen, methylene blue, resveratrol, vitamin A, C, D, E, K.
Gut dysbiosis – direct damage to the microbiome	The goal here is to: • reduce leaky gut by repairing the gut-blood barrier • restore the beneficial microbiome • improve gastroparesis • restore normal bowel movements *Probiotics, *prebiotics, *postbiotics, butyrate, collagen, colostrum, lactoferrin, BPC-157(peptide), KPV (peptide), apigenin, larazotide (peptide), rifaximin (if associated with SIBO), fecal transplant (oral or procedure)
Histamine/MCAS – triggering mast cell degranulation	The goal is to: • stabilize mast cells instead of inhibiting histamine, a more effective treatment. • The main reason is that mast cells have many more substances besides histamine. Cetirizine/cyproheptadine, famotidine, ketotifen, cromolyn, Montelukast, Omalizumab, quercetin, luteolin, EGCG, vitamin D, bromelain, apigenin, resveratrol, honokiol, theanine, kaempferol

***See gut dysbiosis chapter.**

Nicotine Patch

While this remains a potential treatment, please remember that the empirical evidence for its use to treat Long COVID is limited. There is one pilot study involving 4 patients (non-placebo controlled), and there is plenty of **anecdotal evidence** from individual reports that indicate that nicotine patches may help some individuals manage symptoms associated with Long COVID, including fatigue and cognitive impairment. However, rigorous clinical trials are still needed to establish efficacy.

> *"The toxins and oxidants in tobacco counteract any benefit that you could get from nicotine. Do not attempt this using any tobacco products, and this includes vaping."*

Beneficial mechanisms in Long COVID

1. Nicotine activates the *nicotinic acetylcholine receptor* (nAChR), which is responsible for communication between neurons (nerve cells) and involved in almost every synaptic nerve signal transmission. There is a possibility that SARS-CoV-2 binds to these nAChRs on a large scale in a non-intrinsic way, which is a plausible explanation for the widespread symptoms of Long-haul COVID-19. COVID and possibly the spike protein competes for these receptors against the natural Acetylcholine (ACh). Competing prevents cholinergic neuromodulation's normal activation and function at the nicotinic receptors.

2. Nicotine also binds to a subgroup of nAChR called α7-nAChR. This receptor, located primarily on macrophages and nerve cells, is responsible for the cholinergic anti-inflammatory pathway

(CAP). Interestingly, both vagus nerve stimulation and ivermectin may work through this pathway.

3. Nicotine upregulates Angiotensin Converting Enzyme-2 (ACE2) receptor expression on cells. This receptor is on most cells of the body, particularly the epithelial cells of the gut. While SARS-cov-2 uses this receptor to bind, enter, and infect each cell, it also reduces the number of ACE2 receptors each cell has. ACE2 receptors help modulate BP and inflammation. The entire complex gets engulfed in the cell when the virus attaches to the ACE2 receptor through its spike protein. The ACE2 receptor is destroyed and not returned to the surface of the cell. After some time, little to no ACE2 receptors remain on the cell surface. The only way to get the ACE2 receptors back to the cell's surface is to make more. Nicotine activates the genes responsible for creating more ACE2 receptors.

4. Nicotine can increase vagus nerve activity.

5. Nicotine activates the **nicotinic acetylcholine receptor** which decreases **chronic inflammation.**

Nicotine has many negative effects

1. **Endothelial Dysfunction**: Nicotine exposure has been shown to impair endothelial function, which is crucial for maintaining vascular health. **Endothelial dysfunction** can lead to increased vascular permeability and promote inflammation, both of which are key factors in atherosclerosis development. This can promote clots.
2. **Oxidative Stress**: Nicotine increases oxidative stress in vascular tissues, promoting the oxidation of low-density lipoprotein (LDL) cholesterol. Oxidized LDL is a significant contributor to plaque formation in arteries, which is central to atherosclerosis. Nicotine is an **oxidant**!
3. **Platelet Activation**: Nicotine can enhance platelet aggregation, increasing the risk of thrombosis (blood clot formation), which can

further complicate atherosclerotic disease. Besides blood vessel endothelial dysfunction, it promotes clots thru the platelet system. These appear to be limited to smoking and not nicotine patches.

4. **Inflammation**: While nicotine can decrease inflammation by activating the nicotine acetylcholine receptors, it can also promote it as well. Nicotine stimulates the release of pro-inflammatory cytokines and chemokines, exacerbating vascular inflammation. This inflammatory response contributes to the progression of atherosclerotic plaques.
5. Nicotine causes tachycardia (fast heart rate). As a side effect because it is a **stimulant**.
6. Nicotine can worsen insulin resistance, worsening diabetes, and metabolic syndrome.
7. Nicotine can worsen neurodegeneration.
8. Don't forget that nicotine is very addictive.

While there are some benefits, nicotine is a double-edged sword so the line between benefit and risk begins to blur. Even nicotine replacement therapy like nicotine gum and nicotine patches, because they contain nicotine, still are subject to the negative effects. There are many available anti-inflammatory supplements, why choose a risky one?

Negative consequences tend to outweigh the positive so if you decide to use a nicotine patch, keep it very short term, under 30 days. I do not agree with the multi-month and years of continuous or cycling on and off of the nicotine patch use that is being promoted on social media. These negative effects are cumulative and don't reverse when you stop wearing the patch or chewing the nicotine gum. This is why I recommend keeping the treatment time short if you choose to use this method.

References:

1. Leitzke, M. Is the post-COVID-19 syndrome a severe impairment of acetylcholine-orchestrated neuromodulation that responds to

nicotine administration? *Bioelectron Med* **9**, 2 (2023). https://doi.org/10.1186/s42234-023-00104-7

2. South, A. M., Diz, D. I., & Chappell, M. C. (2020). COVID-19, ACE2, and the cardiovascular consequences. *American Journal of Physiology-Heart and Circulatory Physiology, 318*(5), H1084–H1090. https://doi.org/10.1152/ajpheart.00217.2020

3. Maddatu J, Anderson-Baucum E, Evans-Molina C. Smoking and the risk of type 2 diabetes. Transl Res. 2017 Jun;184:101-107. doi: 10.1016/j.trsl.2017.02.004. Epub 2017 Mar 6. PMID: 28336465; PMCID: PMC5429867.

4. Zhang W, Lin H, Zou M, Yuan Q, Huang Z, Pan X, Zhang W. Nicotine in Inflammatory Diseases: Anti-Inflammatory and Pro-Inflammatory Effects. Front Immunol. 2022 Feb 18;13:826889. doi: 10.3389/fimmu.2022.826889. PMID: 35251010; PMCID: PMC8895249.

5. Benowitz NL, Fitzgerald GA, Wilson M, Zhang Q. Nicotine effects on eicosanoid formation and hemostatic function: comparison of transdermal nicotine and cigarette smoking. J Am Coll Cardiol. 1993 Oct;22(4):1159-67. doi: 10.1016/0735-1097(93)90431-y. PMID: 7691912.

Low Dose Naltrexone

Low-Dose Naltrexone (LDN) has been explored as a potential treatment for multiple chronic conditions, including Long COVID, due to its unique pharmacological effects.

1. Modulation of Immune Response

- **Anti-inflammatory Effects:** LDN can minimize inflammation by modulating the immune system. It does so by reducing the production of pro-inflammatory cytokines and increasing anti-inflammatory cytokines, which might help alleviate the chronic inflammatory state seen in Long COVID.

- **Microglial Cell Inhibition:** LDN can inhibit microglial cells in the central nervous system. When overactive, these cells can contribute to neuroinflammation, often manifested in symptoms like brain fog and fatigue in Long COVID.

2. Increase in Endorphins: At low doses, naltrexone temporarily blocks opioid receptors, leading to a rebound effect that enhances the production of endorphins and enkephalins. These endogenous opioids have pain-relieving properties and can improve mood and overall well-being, which might be beneficial for Long COVID patients experiencing chronic pain and mood disturbances.

3. Reduction in Neuropathic Pain: LDN has been reported to help with neuropathic pain, which could be beneficial for Long COVID patients experiencing nerve-related pain or discomfort.

4. Reduction in Fatigue: By modulating immune responses and reducing inflammation, LDN may help improve energy levels and reduce fatigue – one of the most debilitating symptoms of Long COVID.

5. Mitochondrial Assistance

- **Reduction in Inflammation:** Decreased Pro-inflammatory Cytokines: LDN has been demonstrated to reduce the levels of pro-inflammatory cytokines. Chronic inflammation can impair mitochondrial function by increasing oxidative stress and damaging mitochondrial DNA. By reducing inflammation, LDN may help protect mitochondria and enhance their function.
- **Increased Endorphin Levels:** LDN increases the production of endogenous opioids like beta-endorphins, which have been illustrated to have protective effects on cells, including mitochondria. In addition, endorphins can promote cellular repair and reduce oxidative stress.
- **Mitochondrial Biogenesis:** Some evidence suggests that LDN may promote mitochondrial biogenesis—the process by which new mitochondria are formed within cells. It can lead to improved energy production and better cellular function overall.
- **Reduction in Oxidative Stress**: Antioxidant Effects: LDN might have antioxidant characteristics that help reduce oxidative stress, a significant contributor to mitochondrial damage. By lowering oxidative stress, LDN can help maintain mitochondrial integrity and function.

Safety and Side Effects

LDN is generally well-tolerated, but potential side effects can include:

- Sleep disturbances - vivid dreams or insomnia.
- Digestive issues: Mild gastrointestinal symptoms like nausea or constipation.
- Headaches

References:

1. O'Kelly, B., Vidal, L., McHugh, T., Woo, J., Avramovic, G., & Lambert, J. S. (2022). Safety and efficacy of low dose naltrexone in a long COVID cohort: An interventional pre-post study. *Brain, Behavior, & Immunity - Health*, 24, 100485. https://doi.org/10.1016/j.bbih.2022.100485

2. L., et al. (2020). Low Dose Naltrexone: A Review of its Efficacy and Safety Profile. *Journal of Clinical Medicine*.

Guanfacine

Guanfacine—an alpha-2 adrenergic agonist—is primarily used for treating Attention Deficit Hyperactivity Disorder (ADHD) and hypertension. However, its potential benefits for Long COVID are being studied due to its effects on the central nervous system and its ability to modulate the ANS. Here is how *guanfacine* might help in Long COVID:

1. Reduction in Autonomic Dysregulation

Sympathetic Nervous System Modulation: Guanfacine can reduce sympathetic nervous system activity, which may help alleviate symptoms of autonomic dysfunction, such as heart rate variability, dizziness, and blood pressure fluctuations, commonly reported in Long COVID. Patients experiencing symptoms of dysautonomia—such as Postural Orthostatic Tachycardia Syndrome (POTS)—have reported some relief with guanfacine.

2. Neuroprotective Effects

- **Cognitive Benefit:** Guanfacine has been demonstrated to enhance prefrontal cortex function, which is critical for executive functions such as working memory, attention, and cognitive flexibility. It might help with brain fog and cognitive impairments observed in Long COVID patients. Some patients have reported improved attention, memory, and overall cognitive function.

- **Reduction in Neuroinflammation:** By modulating noradrenergic signaling, *guanfacine* may help reduce neuroinflammation, which is believed to contribute to the neurological symptoms of Long COVID.

3. Improvement in Sleep and Anxiety

- **Sedative Effects:** Guanfacine has a mild sedative effect that can help improve sleep quality and reduce anxiety, both of which are commonly impacted in Long COVID patients.

- **Reduction in Hyperarousal:** Guanfacine may help with hyperarousal symptoms by calming the nervous system and better managing Long COVID.

Safety and Side Effects

Guanfacine is generally well-tolerated, but potential **side effects** can include:

- **Sedation:** It creates drowsiness and fatigue, particularly when starting the medication or increasing the dose.

- **Hypotension:** Lowering of BP, which can cause dizziness or lightheadedness.

- **Bradycardia:** Slowing of the heart rate.

- **Dry Mouth:** Common but typically mild.

- **Digestive Issues:** Occasionally causes gastrointestinal symptoms like constipation.

References:

1. Fesharaki-Zadeh, A., Lowe, N., & Arnsten, A. F. T. (2023). Clinical experience with the α2A-adrenoceptor agonist, guanfacine, and N-acetylcysteine for the treatment of cognitive deficits in "Long-COVID19". *Neuroimmunology Reports, 3,* 100154. https://doi.org/10.1016/j.nerep.2022.100154.

Pyridostigmine

Pyridostigmine is an **acetylcholinesterase inhibitor**, meaning it enhances the levels of acetylcholine, a neurotransmitter that plays a crucial role in muscle activation and autonomic nervous system function. In conditions like ME/CFS, where dysautonomia and poor circulation are common, enhancing acetylcholine may improve neurovascular regulation and exercise capacity. It appears to help with **exercise tolerance** when compared to placebo. **Huperzine A**, a supplement, works similarly.

Pyridostigmine is a medication primarily used to treat conditions like **myasthenia gravis**, a neuromuscular disorder, and in some cases, **orthostatic hypotension** and **dysautonomia**, including Postural Orthostatic Tachycardia Syndrome (POTS). It works by inhibiting the enzyme acetylcholinesterase, increasing the amount of acetylcholine available for neuromuscular transmission. However, like all medications, pyridostigmine can cause side effects.

Common Side Effects

These are usually related to its cholinergic action (increased acetylcholine):

1. **Gastrointestinal Issues**
    - **Diarrhea**: Increased motility of the gastrointestinal tract.
    - **Abdominal cramps**: Due to increased smooth muscle activity.
    - **Nausea and vomiting**.
    - **Increased salivation**: Due to stimulation of salivary glands.

2. **Muscle Cramps**
    - Some patients experience muscle twitching or cramps due to overstimulation of neuromuscular junctions.
3. **Increased Urination**
    - Pyridostigmine increases smooth muscle tone in the bladder, leading to more frequent urination.
4. **Sweating**
    - Overstimulation of sweat glands can lead to increased sweating.
5. **Runny Nose (Rhinorrhea)**
    - Cholinergic stimulation can increase nasal secretions.
6. **Bradycardia (Slow Heart Rate)**
    - Pyridostigmine can reduce heart rate by increasing parasympathetic activity.

Less Common/Serious Side Effects

While less common, these side effects can be more serious and may require medical attention:

1. **Muscle Weakness**
    - Paradoxically, excessive doses can cause muscle weakness due to overstimulation of the muscles (cholinergic crisis).
2. **Bronchospasm (Difficulty Breathing)**
    - Overstimulation of bronchial smooth muscle can cause difficulty breathing, which can be serious in patients with respiratory conditions like asthma.
3. **Heart Rhythm Problems**
    - Pyridostigmine can lead to irregular heartbeats or exacerbation of bradycardia in certain individuals.
4. **Severe Abdominal Pain**

- Intense gastrointestinal cramping may sometimes occur and be problematic, particularly in patients with pre-existing gastrointestinal conditions.

5. **Confusion or Cognitive Changes** (Rare)
   - While rare, some patients may experience central nervous system side effects, including confusion or difficulty concentrating, especially if there's cholinergic overload.

Cholinergic Crisis

A **cholinergic crisis** is a severe, life-threatening condition that can occur with an overdose of pyridostigmine.

- **Severe muscle weakness** or paralysis, including respiratory muscles.
- **Extreme bradycardia or hypotension**.
- **Respiratory failure**: Due to bronchoconstriction and muscle weakness.
- **Excessive salivation and sweating**.
- **Blurred vision and difficulty speaking**.

In the case of cholinergic crisis, immediate medical attention is needed, and atropine (an anticholinergic agent) is typically administered as an antidote.

References:

1. Davis HE, McCorkell L, Vogel JM, Topol EJ. Long COVID: major findings, mechanisms and recommendations. Nat Rev Microbiol. 2023 Mar;21(3):133-146. doi: 10.1038/s41579-022-00846-2. Epub 2023 Jan 13. Erratum in: Nat Rev Microbiol. 2023 Jun;21(6):408. doi: 10.1038/s41579-023-00896-0. PMID: 36639608; PMCID: PMC9839201.

2. Joseph P, Pari R, Miller S, Warren A, Stovall MC, Squires J, Chang CJ, Xiao W, Waxman AB, Systrom DM. Neurovascular Dysregulation and Acute Exercise Intolerance in Myalgic Encephalomyelitis/Chronic Fatigue Syndrome: A Randomized, Placebo-Controlled Trial of Pyridostigmine. Chest. 2022 Nov;162(5):1116-1126. doi: 10.1016/j.chest.2022.04.146. Epub 2022 May 6. PMID: 35526605.

3. Squires, J., Al-Zayer, S., & Systrom, D. (2023). Exercise capacity in myalgic encephalomyelitis/chronic fatigue syndrome (ME/CFS) treated with long-term pyridostigmine. *European Respiratory Journal*, *62*(suppl 67), PA4639. https://doi.org/10.1183/13993003.congress-2023.PA4639

Hyperbaric Oxygen Therapy (HBOT)

It has been explored as a potential treatment for Long COVID due to its ability to enhance tissue oxygenation and support the recovery of damaged tissues. The therapy involves breathing pure oxygen in a pressurized environment, which increases the amount of oxygen dissolved in the blood and promotes healing in hypoxic tissues. Due to the potential oxygen toxicity, if you will do these treatments, pair them with before and after oral antioxidants.

Mechanism of Action for Long COVID

1. **Tissue Oxygenation**: HBOT significantly increases oxygen delivery to tissues, which can aid in repairing damage caused by prolonged hypoxia (low oxygen levels), a condition seen in severe COVID-19 cases and sometimes persisting in Long COVID. This can improve cellular metabolism and energy production, especially in tissues where oxygen supply has been compromised.

2. **Reduction of Inflammation**: HBOT has anti-inflammatory properties and can decrease systemic inflammation, which is elevated in many Long COVID patients. It helps modulate the release of pro-inflammatory cytokines like IL-6 and TNF-α, both of which are associated with persistent inflammatory responses in Long COVID.

3. **Neurological and Cognitive Support**: HBOT has been used in treating conditions like traumatic brain injury and stroke, and similar mechanisms might be beneficial in Long COVID patients suffering from cognitive issues like "brain fog." The therapy promotes neurogenesis (the creation of new neurons) and

enhances brain oxygenation, potentially aiding in cognitive recovery.

4. **Mitochondrial Function**: HBOT may also improve mitochondrial function, which is essential in managing the energy-related issues experienced by Long COVID patients, such as chronic fatigue. Oxygen helps support mitochondrial energy production through oxidative phosphorylation, which can be impaired in Long COVID.

Clinical Evidence

- A **2022 randomized controlled trial** conducted in Israel demonstrated that HBOT improved cognitive function, energy levels, and respiratory symptoms in Long COVID patients compared to a placebo group. The study reported a significant improvement in memory, attention, and executive function, as well as a reduction in persistent fatigue.

- Another **2021 study** found that HBOT improved cardiovascular function and oxygen saturation levels in patients who had experienced moderate to severe COVID-19, suggesting that the therapy might help reduce post-COVID-19 complications.

Risks and Limitations

While HBOT has shown promise, it is not without risks. The therapy can cause **barotrauma** (damage to the ears or lungs due to pressure changes) and **oxygen toxicity**, especially with long-term or improper use. These risks need to be carefully managed in clinical settings.

Conclusion

HBOT offers a potential therapeutic approach for Long COVID, particularly for patients with persistent hypoxia, inflammation, cognitive dysfunction, and fatigue. However, more large-scale studies are required to confirm its efficacy and to better understand which patients may benefit the most from the treatment.

References:

- Robbins, T., et al. (2022). *The use of hyperbaric oxygen therapy for long COVID: A prospective randomized controlled study*. Frontiers in Medicine, 9.

- Zilberman-Itskovich, S., et al. (2021). *Hyperbaric oxygen therapy improves cognitive function and symptoms in long COVID patients*. The Lancet.

Clots, Coagulation, and Blood thinners

Why is Clotting Included in a Long COVID book?

Long COVID causes abnormal and pathological clots to form for several reasons. These clots can cause heart attacks, strokes, clots to form in your legs such as deep vein thrombosis (DVT) which can embolize or migrate into the lungs blood vessels causing a pulmonary embolus (PE). Unfortunately, all of these have a potential to be fatal.

What is the Purpose of Blood Clots?

Clots do serve an important purpose in our bodies. This may seem like an obvious answer, and it is. The primary purpose of **clots** and the **clotting process** (also known as **coagulation**) is to prevent **excessive bleeding** and promote **wound healing** after an injury. Clotting is a critical mechanism for maintaining **hemostasis**, which is the balance between bleeding and clot formation. Being able to clot is essential to survival.

The point of clots is to stop blood flow. Clots are inherently stable and are meant to stop blood flow until the injury causing the bleeding is repaired. Clots <u>do not</u> dissolve on their own, they need help using a natural clot dissolving system called plasmin. When a large clot forms, it can completely obstruct blood flow. While that needs to happen to allow repair, sometimes the clotting cascade and mechanism is triggered due to an abnormal reason. Clots do serve a very important purpose. Stopping the blood flow or reduction of blood flow can cause **ischemia** (the organ is starving for oxygen) or **infarct** (the organ area dies off). Clots don't just come and go.

- **Preventing blood loss**
  - When a blood vessel is injured, the clotting process forms a **blood clot** to **seal the damaged area**, stopping further **bleeding** (hemorrhage). This prevents excessive blood loss and helps maintain **circulatory stability**.
- **Sealing wounds**
  - Clots help **plug** the injury site in the blood vessel, acting as a temporary seal. This gives time for the underlying **tissue repair mechanisms** to take over, enabling the damaged vessel and tissues to heal.
- **Providing a scaffold for tissue repair**
  - The clot serves as a **framework** for the migration of cells like **fibroblasts** and **endothelial cells**, which are involved in wound healing. This leads to the formation of new tissue and blood vessels at the injury site.
- **Preventing infection**
  - By sealing the wound, blood clots act as a **barrier** against pathogens such as **bacteria** or **viruses**, reducing the risk of infection at the injury site.
- **Restoring blood vessel integrity**
  - Once a clot forms and stabilizes the area, the body can begin repairing the blood vessel walls. Over time, the clot will be dissolved through **fibrinolysis**, and normal blood flow will be restored.
- **Maintaining vascular health**
  - The clotting system also helps regulate vascular health by balancing **pro-coagulant** and **anti-coagulant** factors. This balance prevents both **uncontrolled bleeding** and the formation of unnecessary clots (which can lead to conditions like **thrombosis**).

Clot Resolution

- For the purposes listed above, the clot needs to be physically and actively broken down (**fibrinolysis** or **thrombolysis**) and removed to allow for blood flow to resume once the blood vessel is repaired. Clots do not break down on their own, they are broken down using an active process. Clots are broken down using our own plasmin system.

Plasminogen and Plasmin

- **Plasminogen**: Plasmin is derived from its inactive precursor, plasminogen, which is incorporated into a blood clot during its formation. Plasminogen circulates in the bloodstream and is produced primarily by the liver.

- **Activation**: Plasminogen is activated to plasmin through several mechanisms, primarily involving tissue plasminogen activator (tPA), which is released from endothelial cells, especially in response to vascular injury or thrombus formation. Other activators include urokinase and streptokinase.

Blood Thinners

Although commonly grouped under one name, the different types of categories work in very different ways to affect the clotting system. All of these are considered "blood thinners". The term "blood thinners" It is a bit of a misnomer, as anticoagulants don't actually thin the blood. Instead, they work by inhibiting the blood's ability to clot. The name likely originated from the observable effect these medications have on the blood's viscosity and the overall flow. When clotting is reduced, the blood can flow more freely, leading to the perception that the blood is "thinner."

The use of the term became popular in medical settings and among the public because it's easier to understand than the more technical terms like "anticoagulants" or "antithrombotic agents." While the terminology can be misleading, it effectively communicates the intended outcome of these medications, which is to prevent harmful clots.

It refers to the following agents

- **antiplatelet agents** – inhibit platelet function.
- **fibrinolytics (thrombolytics)** – break clots apart by attacking fibrin.
- **anticoagulants** – prevents clots from forming. Inhibit clotting factors.

These medications are essential when blood clots form abnormally, often due to pathological conditions. For instance, **damage to the endothelial lining** of blood vessels can trigger clot formation, or **abnormal proteins** circulating in the bloodstream can activate the intrinsic clotting pathway. In these situations, the body's natural balance is disrupted, increasing the likelihood of inappropriate clotting. The medications act to restore this balance by preventing clot formation, dissolving clots, or inhibiting platelet function.

Antiplatelet Agents

Prevent Platelet Function or Aggregation.

These drugs reduce the ability of platelets to stick together (aggregate), thus preventing the formation of a blood clot.

Common Antiplatelet Drugs

- **Aspirin**: Inhibits the enzyme cyclooxygenase (COX), preventing thromboxane A2 formation, a potent platelet activator.
- **Clopidogrel (Plavix)**: Blocks the P2Y12 receptor on platelets, reducing activation.
- **Prasugrel (Effient)**: Similar to clopidogrel but has a more potent effect on the P2Y12 receptor.
- **Ticagrelor (Brilinta)**: A reversible P2Y12 inhibitor with faster onset.
- **Dipyridamole**: Increases cyclic AMP in platelets, inhibiting aggregation.

- **NSAIDs**: Non-steroidal anti-inflammatory drugs, although primarily used for pain, can have blood-thinning effects similar to aspirin.
- **Abciximab (ReoPro)**: A glycoprotein IIb/IIIa inhibitor, preventing platelets from binding fibrinogen; no longer available in the USA due to production issues.

Anticoagulants

Prevent Clotting Factor Cascade Progression.

Anticoagulants interfere with the cascade of clotting factors that lead to clot formation. They are key for preventing clots in at-risk patients.

Common Anticoagulant Drugs

- **Heparin**: Enhances antithrombin III, which inactivates thrombin and other clotting factors (Factors IIa, IXa, Xa).
- **Warfarin**: A vitamin K antagonist, inhibiting the synthesis of clotting factors II, VII, IX, and X in the liver.
- **Apixaban (Eliquis)**: Directly inhibits Factor Xa, preventing clot formation.
- **Rivaroxaban (Xarelto)**: Another direct Factor Xa inhibitor.
- **Dabigatran (Pradaxa)**: Directly inhibits thrombin (Factor IIa).
- **Edoxaban (Lixiana)**: Direct Xa inhibitor.
- **Betrixaban (Bevyxxa)**: Direct Xa inhibitor, recently withdrawn from the market (not due to safety concerns).

Fibrinolytic Agents (Thrombolytics)

Dissolve Existing Clots.

Fibrinolytic drugs activate the plasminogen system, converting plasminogen to plasmin, which breaks down fibrin clots. Unlike anticoagulants, <u>they do not prevent clot formation</u>. These are often used in acute settings, such as during a heart attack or stroke, and are administered intravenously.

Common Fibrinolytic Agents

- **Anistreplase**: Activates plasminogen and promotes clot breakdown.
- **Desmoteplase**: Derived from the saliva of vampire bats, used for thrombolysis.
- **Streptokinase**: (Not to be confused with **Serra** starting fibrinolytics that come from silkworms) produced by Streptococci bacteria, activates plasminogen. Overdose can be reversed using **aminocaproic acid.**
- **Tissue Plasminogen Activator (tPA)**: A synthetic version of a natural clot-dissolving enzyme.

Over-the-Counter (OTC) Fibrinolytics
These naturally derived substances support **mild fibrinolysis** and are available as supplements. These do not work in the same capacity as intravenous fibrinolytics and would otherwise no be considered safe to be offered over the counter.

- **Serrapeptase (Serratiopeptidase)**
  - **Origin**: Serrapeptase is produced by the bacterium *Serratia* found in the digestive system of silkworms.
  - **Type of Protease**: It is a serine protease, which means it breaks down proteins through a **serine amino acid** at its active site.
  - **Fibrinolytic Properties**: Serrapeptase is known for its anti-inflammatory and fibrinolytic (clot-dissolving) properties. It helps break down fibrin, the protein involved in blood clotting, and promotes the clearance of debris from inflamed areas, thereby supporting tissue repair. It is often used for its ability to reduce inflammation and promote healing by breaking down non-living tissue.

- **Nattokinase**
  - **Origin**: Nattokinase is derived from *Natto*, a traditional Japanese food made from fermented soybeans, where the enzyme is produced by the bacterium *Bacillus subtilis* during fermentation.
  - **Type of Protease**: serine protease
  - **Fibrinolytic Properties**: Nattokinase exhibits potent fibrinolytic activity by directly breaking down fibrin, and it has been shown to enhance the body's own production of plasmin (the primary enzyme responsible for breaking down blood clots). Nattokinase can also reduce levels of clotting factors such as fibrinogen, Factor VII, and Factor VIII , contributing to its anticoagulant effects.
- **Lumbrokinase**
  - **Origin**: Lumbrokinase comes from earthworms, particularly the *Lumbricus rubellus* species.
  - **Type of Protease**: serine proteases
  - **Fibrinolytic Properties**: It is highly effective at breaking down fibrin and promoting blood clot dissolution. Lumbrokinase has been used in traditional Chinese medicine for its ability to treat thrombotic diseases, reduce blood viscosity, and prevent clot formation, making it an option for cardiovascular health.
- **Bromelain**
  - **Origin**: Bromelain is extracted from pineapples, particularly the stem and fruit.
  - **Type of Protease**: cysteine protease
  - **Fibrinolytic Properties**: Bromelain has a wide range of therapeutic uses, including anti-inflammatory, anti-edematous, and fibrinolytic effects. It works by enhancing the degradation of fibrin and other protein complexes associated

with clot formation, promoting circulation and reducing swelling. It also inhibits platelet aggregation, reducing the risk of clot formation.

- **Papain**
    - **Origin**: Derived from papaya (from the fruit and leaves).
    - **Type of Protease**: Cysteine protease.
    - **Fibrinolytic Properties**: Helps break down proteins and has mild fibrinolytic properties. It's less potent than serrapeptase or nattokinase for clot dissolution but is still used for its ability to digest proteins and support wound healing.

Comparison

- **Serrapeptase, nattokinase**, and **lumbrokinase** are the most potent in breaking down fibrin and have a strong focus on reducing clot formation and enhancing circulation.
- **Bromelain** and **papain** are effective for mild fibrinolytic action and inflammation reduction but are more well-known for their digestive and anti-inflammatory benefits. They are not really used for fibrinolysis.

H.E.L.P Apheresis (Heparin-induced Extracorporeal LDL Precipitation)

- **Mechanism**: HELP apheresis specifically removes **low-density lipoprotein (LDL)** cholesterol, **lipoprotein(a)** [Lp(a)], and **fibrinogen** from the blood by using **heparin** to precipitate these molecules. Fibrinogen is the main way that HELP apheresis reduces the risk of clotting. It reduces one of the clotting factors.
- **Process**: Blood is drawn from the patient and mixed with heparin, which causes LDL, Lp(a), and fibrinogen to precipitate. These precipitated substances are then removed through filtration, and the remaining blood is returned to the patient.

- **Primary Use**: HELP apheresis is primarily used to treat patients with **familial hypercholesterolemia**, particularly those who do not respond to standard lipid-lowering therapies like statins. It is also used for patients with high **Lipoprotein(a)** or **Lp(a)** levels and certain forms of **atherosclerosis**.
- HELP apheresis does not remove clots, microclots, or spike proteins.
- **Targeted Substances**: LDL cholesterol, Lp(a), fibrinogen. Notice spike proteins and microclots are not listed.

Clotting Cascade Pathways

The clotting system involves two pathways that activate the clotting cascade, leading to the formation of a stable clot.

- **Intrinsic Pathway**
    - Activated by trauma to blood vessels. This can be caused by a ruptured atherosclerosis plaque or damage to the internal blood vessel endothelium (internal lining).
    - Measured by Activated Partial Thromboplastin Time (APTT).
    - Involves factors XII, XI, IX, VIII, X, V, II.
- **Extrinsic Pathway**
    - Triggered by external tissue injury.
    - Measured by Prothrombin Time (PT).
    - Involves factors VII, X, V, and II.

The clotting system is based on checks and balances. Clots are required, but also inappropriate clotting can cause problems.

Antithrombin III (ATIII)

is a naturally occurring anticoagulant protein that plays a crucial role in regulating blood clotting. It is a **serine protease inhibitor** (serpin) that **primarily inhibits thrombin (factor IIa**) and **factor Xa,** along with other proteases in the coagulation cascade like factors IXa, XIa, and XIIa. By inhibiting these clotting factors, antithrombin helps maintain the balance between clot formation and dissolution, preventing excessive clotting (thrombosis).

- **Inhibition of Thrombin and Factor Xa**: Antithrombin binds to thrombin and factor Xa, neutralizing their activity and preventing further conversion of fibrinogen into fibrin, a key component of blood clots. This action helps modulate the coagulation process and keep it under control.

- **Heparin Co-factor**: The activity of antithrombin is significantly enhanced by heparin, a glycosaminoglycan found on the endothelial cells of blood vessels or administered therapeutically. When heparin binds to antithrombin, it induces a conformational change that accelerates its inhibitory activity by 1,000-fold, making it an essential part of heparin's anticoagulant effect.

- **Regulating Blood Clotting**: Antithrombin acts as a natural check on the coagulation system, ensuring that blood clots form only when necessary and that they don't extend excessively. Deficiency in antithrombin, whether inherited or acquired, can result in a hypercoagulable state, leading to an increased risk of thrombosis.

Clinical Relevance

- **Antithrombin Deficiency**: Both congenital and acquired deficiencies of antithrombin can lead to an increased risk of venous thromboembolism (VTE). Acquired deficiency may occur in settings like liver disease, nephrotic syndrome, disseminated intravascular coagulation (DIC), and during prolonged use of heparin (heparin resistance).

- **Therapeutic Use**: In certain clinical situations, antithrombin concentrates may be administered to patients with antithrombin deficiency to reduce the risk of clot formation. These concentrates are often used during surgeries or other high-risk situations for thrombosis.

- **Heparin Resistance**: Some patients may exhibit resistance to heparin therapy, particularly those with low levels of antithrombin. In such cases, supplementing with antithrombin concentrate can restore the effectiveness of heparin.

Negative Consequences of Deficiency

- **Venous Thrombosis**: Antithrombin deficiency is associated with an increased risk of developing venous thrombosis, including deep vein thrombosis (DVT) and pulmonary embolism (PE).

- **Hereditary Antithrombin Deficiency**: This is an autosomal dominant condition where patients are at a lifelong risk of thromboembolic events. Management often involves anticoagulation therapy.

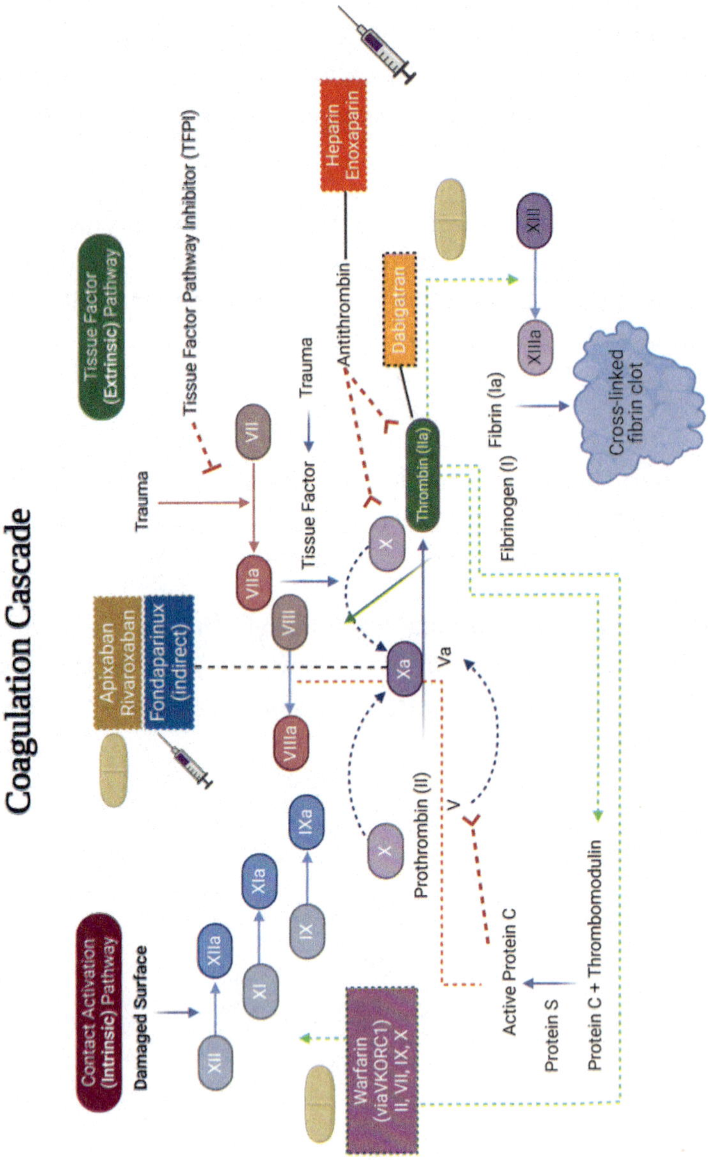

Coagulation Cascade
Contact Activation (Intrinsic) Pathway
Tissue Factor (Extrinsic) Pathway
Damaged Surface
XII
XIIa
XI
XIa
IX
IXa
Trauma
VII
VIIa
Tissue Factor Pathway Inhibitor (TFPI)
Tissue Factor
Trauma
Apixaban
Rivaroxaban
Fondaparinux (indirect)
VIII
VIIIa
X
Xa
X
Va
V
Prothrombin (II)
Thrombin (IIa)
Antithrombin
Heparin
Enoxaparin
Dabigatran
Fibrinogen (I)
Fibrin (Ia)
XIII
XIIIa
Cross-linked fibrin clot
Warfarin (viaVKORC1) II, VII, IX, X
Active Protein C
Protein S
Protein C + Thrombomodulin

Risk Factors for Clotting and Bleeding

- **Increased Risk of Clots**
- **Factor V Leiden**: Mutation leading to excessive clotting.
- **Antiphospholipid Syndrome (aPL)**: Increased the chance of abnormal clot formation.
- **Antiphospholipid Syndrome (APS)**: An autoimmune disorder where the body produces antibodies (anticardiolipin, lupus anticoagulant) that increase clotting risk. It is linked to recurrent miscarriages and deep vein thrombosis (DVT)
- **Protein C:** natural anticoagulant that inactivates clotting factors. Deficiency leads to excessive clotting. Breaks down activated clotting factors like Va and VIIIa, as seen in the figure above.
- **Protein S:** Protein S works with Protein C to inactivate clotting factors. Deficiency increases clot risk. Breaks down activated clotting factors like Va and VIIIa.
- **Antithrombin III Deficiency**: Natural anticoagulants in the blood, and their deficiencies lead to an increased risk of clots.
- **Homocysteine**: Elevated levels linked to endothelial damage and clot formation; influenced by B-vitamin levels.
    - **Elevated Homocysteine Levels**: High levels of homocysteine can damage the endothelium (the inner lining of blood vessels), leading to increased inflammation and promoting the formation of blood clots. It may also increase the expression of tissue factor, a pro-coagulant protein that triggers the clotting cascade.
    - **Nutritional Deficiencies**: Deficiencies in vitamins B6, B12, and folate (Vitamin B9) can contribute to elevated homocysteine levels since these vitamins are essential for its metabolism. Supplementing with these vitamins can help lower homocysteine levels and potentially reduce the risk of clot formation.

- **Plasminogen Activator Inhibitor-1 (PAI-1)** is a protein that plays a key role in regulating blood clotting by inhibiting fibrinolysis, the process that breaks down clots. In normal circumstances, PAI-1 helps maintain a balance between clot formation and breakdown to prevent excessive bleeding or clotting. However, elevated levels of PAI-1 can lead to a higher risk of developing blood clots.

    - **PAI-1 in Long COVID**

        - In the context of Long COVID, PAI-1 has been implicated in various symptoms and complications, especially those related to the cardiovascular and clotting systems.
        - **Chronic Inflammation and Endothelial Dysfunction**: Long COVID is often associated with ongoing inflammation and damage to the endothelial cells that line blood vessels. This inflammation can lead to the overproduction of PAI-1, contributing to impaired fibrinolysis, which may result in excessive clotting in blood vessels.
        - **Hypercoagulability**: Elevated PAI-1 levels can cause a hypercoagulable state, where the blood has a higher tendency to clot. This is seen in some Long COVID patients, leading to increased risks of thrombotic events, such as deep vein thrombosis (DVT) or pulmonary embolism. Microclots in small vessels have also been suggested as a potential cause of some of the persistent symptoms in Long COVID, like fatigue and brain fog.
        - **Tissue Hypoxia**: Due to the formation of clots and the reduced breakdown of these clots (due to high PAI-1 levels), tissues may receive less oxygen. This could be one of the reasons why patients experience symptoms like fatigue, muscle pain, and shortness of breath in Long COVID.
        - **Metabolic Dysregulation**: PAI-1 is also associated with metabolic conditions such as obesity and diabetes, which are risk factors for severe COVID-19 and Long COVID.

Increased PAI-1 levels in these patients may contribute to the persistence of symptoms and complications like insulin resistance or cardiovascular issues.

- **Treatments Targeting PAI-1**

  - Efforts to manage elevated PAI-1 levels in Long COVID might include:
  - **Anticoagulants**: To reduce the risk of excessive clotting, some Long COVID patients may be prescribed blood thinners.
  - **Anti-inflammatory treatments**: By targeting the underlying inflammation, PAI-1 levels could potentially be reduced.
  - **Lifestyle modifications**: Exercise, diet, and managing comorbid conditions like obesity or diabetes can help regulate PAI-1 levels.

Clotting Factors

The clotting cascade is a complex process involving 12 factors plus numerous other proteins, each with a unique role in coagulation.

1. **Factor I (1)** = Fibrinogen *
2. **Factor II (2)** = Prothrombin *
3. **Factor III (3)** = Tissue Factor
4. **Factor IV (4)** = Calcium
5. **Factor V (5)** = Proaccelerin *
6. **Factor VII (7)** = Proconvertin *
7. **Factor VIII (8)** = Antihemophilic Factor *
8. **Factor IX (9)** = Christmas Factor *
9. **Factor X (10)** = Stuart-Prower Factor *
10. **Factor XI (11)** = Plasma Thromboplastin Antecedent *

11. **Factor XII (12)** = Hageman Factor
12. **Factor XIII (13)** = Fibrin Stabilizing Factor *

Liver makes the factors labeled with *. The **liver** is responsible for the manufacturing factors I, II, V, VII, VIII, IX, X, XI, XIII and **protein C** and **protein S**. Also, **Antithrombin III (AT III)** and **plasminogen/plasmin** are made in the liver. **Normal liver function,** is therefore, important for proper clotting system function.

Von Willebrand Factor (vWF), made inside blood vessel endothelium, carries Factor VIII (8). Without vWF, factor VIII rapidly degrades. A deficiency of vWF result in bleeding.

Extrinsic Pathway

1. This IS the major clotting pathway. This is what the clotting mechanism was meant to do: Stop you from bleeding to death after trauma. This pathway is NOT involved in Long COVID because Long COVID doesn't cause physical trauma. Long COVID causes **intrinsic pathway** activation.
2. **Trigger**: The extrinsic pathway is activated by external trauma, such as a cut or injury that leads to bleeding. It responds quickly to more severe injuries. This pathway is meant to stop bleeding from trauma.
3. **Mechanism**: The key player in this pathway is **Tissue Factor (TF),** a protein that is exposed when tissues are injured. When Factor VII (7) contacts tissue factor, it is activated. TF is present in every tissue. Whenever any physical damage occurs to anything like skin, muscle, connective tissues, nerves, etc., TF is exposed and that is what sets off this clotting pathway. When blood comes into contact with TF, it activates Factor VII.
4. **Sequence of Events**
    1. Tissue Factor binds with Factor VII.
    2. This complex activates Factor VII to VIIa.

3. Factor VIIa then activates Factor X, leading to the common pathway of coagulation.

5. **Role**: The extrinsic pathway provides a rapid response to injury and is crucial for initiating clotting immediately after trauma.

Intrinsic Pathway

1. In the context of **Long COVID**, activation of the **intrinsic pathway** of coagulation can occur due to **vascular inflammation** and **endothelial damage**, which are common features of the condition. There are multiple reasons for this.

2. This is an assistant pathway for trauma. It's meant to help the extrinsic pathway in traumatic injuries. However, when it is involved on its own, its due to pathological processes listed below.

3. **Trigger**: This pathway is activated by **damage to the blood vessel wall (vascular endothelium)**. Tissue Factor (TF) exposure is <u>not</u> necessary. This damage can occur spontaneously or due to conditions like atherosclerosis with plaque rupture inside a blood vessel.

4. **Mechanism**: The intrinsic pathway is initiated when blood comes into contact with negatively charged surfaces, such as exposed collagen from damaged endothelial cells. This process involves several clotting factors, primarily factors XII (Hageman factor), XI, IX, and VIII.

5. **Sequence of Events**:

    1. Factor XII activates upon <u>contact with collagen</u>.
    2. Factor XIIa activates Factor XI.
    3. Factor XIa activates Factor IX.
    4. Factor IXa, in the presence of **Factor VIIIa**, activates Factor X.

6. **Role**: This pathway is crucial for amplifying the coagulation response and is particularly important for forming stable clots in response to smaller, localized injuries. Pathologically, its involved for the formation of most of the "bad" type of clots.

1. **Endothelial dysfunction**

   - **Long COVID** has been associated with chronic inflammation of the blood vessels, leading to damage of the **endothelial lining**. This can expose subendothelial components, such as **collagen**, activating the intrinsic pathway.

2. **Microvascular clotting**

   - This is a possible mechanism; however, there is insufficient evidence to support anticoagulant or fibrinolytic treatment at the time of this writing for microclots; it is too early to tell if these have any clinical significance. It is mentioned here because many are currently getting treated for microclots. **Microthrombi** and **persistent coagulopathies** (such as platelet hyperactivation and impaired fibrinolysis) observed in some Long COVID patients can trigger the intrinsic pathway.

   - Tests such as **thrombin generation assays (TGA)** and specific markers of thrombin formation. **Biomarkers** like elevated **Factor XIIa** or **prekallikrein activation** can also indicate intrinsic pathway activation in clinical and research settings.

3. **Chronic inflammation**

   - Ongoing **systemic inflammation** in Long COVID, characterized by elevated levels of pro-inflammatory cytokines, can lead to a **hypercoagulable state**. This inflammation can increase clotting activity by activating intrinsic factors.

4. **Autoimmune mechanisms**

    - Long COVID has been associated with **autoimmune responses** that can damage blood vessels. Autoimmune attacks on endothelial cells may lead to clot formation through intrinsic pathway activation, similar to conditions like **antiphospholipid syndrome**.

Integration of Pathways

Both pathways converge on **Factor X (10)**, where they combine to form the common pathway of coagulation. From this point, it doesn't matter which pathway triggered the cascade, Factor X is activated to Xa, which, along with Factor Va, converts prothrombin to thrombin. **Thrombin** then converts **fibrinogen** to **fibrin**, forming the mesh that constitutes the blood clot.

Both pathways are essential for effective hemostasis (stopping bleeding) and work together to ensure proper clot formation and stability.

Testing for Clotting Disorders

- **Here is what I test for if I suspect clotting to be an issue:**
    - **Antiphospholipid Syndrome (aPL):** Increases are linked to abnormal clot formation.
    - **Antiphospholipid Syndrome (APS)**: Increases are linked to abnormal clot formation.
    - **Protein C:** Deficiency leads to excessive clotting. If the Protein C resistance test suggests **Factor V Leiden** (a mutation of factor 5), a specific genetic test (PCR-based) is performed to identify the presence of the Factor V Leiden mutation (specifically, a mutation in the F5 gene).
    - **Protein S:** Deficiency increases clot risk.

  - **Antithrombin III Deficiency**: deficiency leads to an increased risk of clots.

- **Homocysteine**: Elevated levels linked to endothelial damage and clot
- **In one study (**Taquet 2023), elevated levels of fibrinogen and D-dimer were associated with brain fog.

Reversal Agents

- These are meant to reverse fibrinolytics or break down clots.
- **Tranexamic Acid (TXA)**: Inhibits plasminogen activation, reducing fibrinolysis, used to stop excessive bleeding.
- **Vitamin K**: Reverses the effects of warfarin.
- **Andexanet Alfa**: Reverses the effects of direct Factor Xa inhibitors like apixaban and rivaroxaban.

Microclots vs Microthrombi

Just about everyone with Long COVID has heard about **microclots**. Microclots as described in Long COVID are not the same as regular clots, even microthrombi formed from the clotting factors as listed above. Microclots refer to microscopic clots that are formed from fibrin-amyloid complexes. There are different from microthrombi that are formed from traditional fibrin only complexes. Unfortunately, microclots and microthrombi are being used interchangeably, but they are not.

Why does it matter what they are called?

Microclot-amyloid complexes are resistant to fibrinolytic break down. Traditional clot microthrombi are not.

So, what exactly are microclots?

Microclots are not the same as microthrombi as mentioned above, (small clots in small blood vessels). Microclots, as the term is used with Long COVID, are complexes that form with amyloid proteins. Fibrin is mixed together with amyloid proteins. These make these microclots very resistant to breakdown by the plasmin system. Even fibrinolytics have a difficult time to break these down. They would certainly not break down on their own. Microclots don't cause your hands or feet to turn purple or red or white and then go back to normal. We just said that they don't break down easily or on their own. If a traditional microthrombi stops blood flow, that area will undergo a process called **ischemia** (starving for oxygen but gets a bit) followed by **gangrene** (dying) and **necrosis** (died off). The area will turn black. That is what happens when oxygenated blood flow is stopped to an area for any prolonged amount of time. How many Long Covid patients have you heard of with microclots are losing toes and fingers?

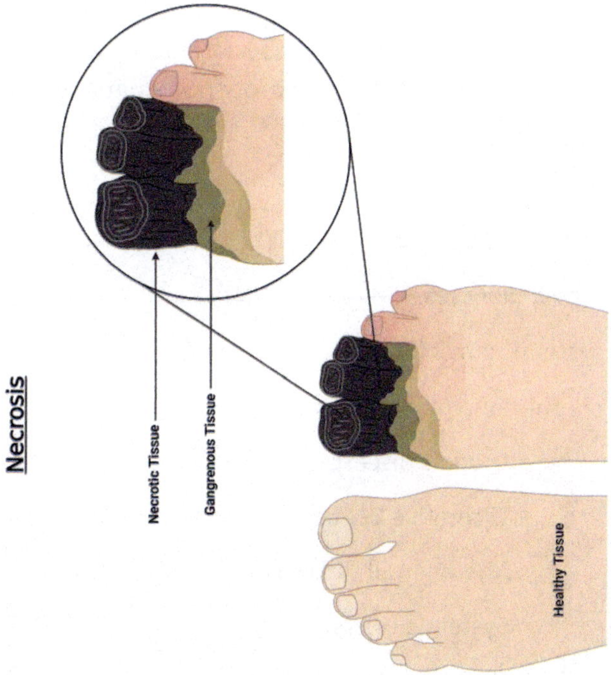

Where do the amyloid proteins come from?

Most of these are still hypotheses.

1. One is that structure fibrinogen is altered.
2. Another is that amyloid fibrils are formed from misfolded proteins from oxidative stress, tissue damage, of inflammation.
3. Lastly, it is the spike protein interaction with fibrinogen.

What are microclots made of and why do they occur?

Altered fibrin proteins together with amyloid like fibrils that can form these breakdown resistant amyloid-fibrin complexes that have been called microclots.

Microclots with amyloid complexes are not new and have been seen for years using the same tools that are used for Long COVID. It involves using a fluorogenic amyloid stain and using a special microscope. Each and every one of the diseases listed below have been documented to also form amyloid-like fibrin clots:

- Alzheimer's
- Parkinson's disease
- type 2 diabetes
- systemic amyloidosis
- chronic inflammatory conditions
    - Crohn's disease
    - Ulcerative Colitis
    - Rheumatoid Arthritis
    - Systemic Lupus
    - Chronic kidney disease
    - atherosclerosis
    - Long COVID

- While these clots contribute to disease pathology, treatments primarily focus on other aspects of the disease and the microclots themselves are not typically targeted for direct treatment. Why is that? Why don't we treat any of these diseases with antiplatelet, anticoagulants, or fibrinolytics?

What is Plasminogen activator inhibitor 1 (PAI-1)?

PAI-1 is a protein that regulates blood clotting and other processes. PAI-1 inhibits the action of plasminogen activators that convert plasminogen to plasmin. In basic terms, it prevents plasminogen from activating to plasmin so it prevents clot breakdown.

Is a PAI-1 mutation involved?

I see tests for PAI-1 being ordered routinely. PAI-1 has been implicated to microclots. PAI-1 deficiency is a rare inherited autosomal recessive bleeding disorder characterized by too much breakdown of clots leading to a lifelong moderate bleeding disorder. So, mutations of this gene are not relevant then to Long COVID.

What about elevated levels of PAI-1?

Elevated levels of **plasminogen activator inhibitor-1 (PAI-1)** can result from various physiological and pathological factors and are not specific to Long COVID. PAI-1 is a key regulator of fibrinolysis, inhibiting tissue plasminogen activator (tPA) and urokinase (uPA), and its overexpression can increase the risk of thrombosis and cardiovascular disease. Increased PPA-1 can be caused by chronic inflammation. **In short, elevated levels of PAI-1** can lead to a higher risk of developing blood clots. If the **PAI-1 elevated**, it will inhibit the plasmin clot breakdown system and it makes sense to at least to consider:

- **Anticoagulants**: To reduce the risk of excessive clotting, some Long COVID patients may be prescribed blood thinners.
- **Anti-inflammatory treatments**: By targeting the underlying inflammation, PAI-1 levels could potentially be reduced.

- **Lifestyle modifications**: Exercise, diet, and managing comorbid conditions like obesity or diabetes can help regulate PAI-1 levels.

What causes PAI-1 increases?

1. Obesity and Metabolic Syndrome

- **Mechanism**: PAI-1 levels are often elevated in individuals with obesity, particularly those with central adiposity. Adipose tissue itself can produce PAI-1, contributing to increased levels in circulation. This elevation is linked to metabolic syndrome, characterized by insulin resistance, hypertension, and dyslipidemia.

- **Implications**: Obesity-induced PAI-1 elevation increases the risk of cardiovascular diseases and type 2 diabetes.

2. Insulin Resistance and Type 2 Diabetes

- **Mechanism**: Hyperinsulinemia, often observed in insulin resistance and type 2 diabetes, stimulates the production of PAI-1. Elevated PAI-1 can impair fibrinolysis, increasing the risk of atherosclerosis and other cardiovascular complications in these patients.

- **Studies**: Research shows that insulin resistance is positively correlated with increased PAI-1 levels in both type 2 diabetics and individuals with metabolic syndrome.

3. Inflammation and Infection

- **Mechanism**: Inflammatory cytokines, such as tumor necrosis factor-alpha (TNF-α) and interleukin-6 (IL-6), can upregulate PAI-1 production. These cytokines are commonly elevated during chronic inflammation, autoimmune disorders, or acute infections.

- **Conditions**: Sepsis and chronic inflammatory diseases such as rheumatoid arthritis and lupus are associated with elevated PAI-1 levels due to persistent inflammation.

4. Aging

- **Mechanism**: Aging is associated with an increase in circulating PAI-1 levels, potentially due to chronic low-grade inflammation, known as "inflammaging," and the gradual loss of insulin sensitivity over time.

- **Clinical Relevance**: Higher PAI-1 in older individuals contributes to increased cardiovascular risk, including atherosclerosis and stroke.

5. Cardiovascular Disease and Atherosclerosis

- **Mechanism**: Elevated PAI-1 is both a consequence and a driver of cardiovascular disease. It can contribute to the development and progression of atherosclerotic plaques by inhibiting fibrinolysis, thus promoting clot formation and plaque stability.

- **Clinical Evidence**: Elevated PAI-1 is often found in patients with coronary artery disease and is associated with an increased risk of myocardial infarction and stroke.

6. Hormonal Imbalances

- **Mechanism**: Elevated levels of certain hormones like **glucocorticoids** and **estrogens** can lead to higher PAI-1 levels. Cortisol, which is released during stress or as a response to exogenous corticosteroid treatment, can induce PAI-1 expression. Additionally, the hormonal changes during pregnancy can increase PAI-1 levels, which normalizes postpartum.

- **Examples**: Corticosteroid therapy and conditions like Cushing's syndrome are linked to higher PAI-1 levels.

7. Genetics

- **Mechanism**: Genetic polymorphisms in the PAI-1 gene, such as the 4G/5G polymorphism, can lead to higher expression of PAI-1. Individuals with the 4G allele are predisposed to elevated PAI-1 levels, increasing their risk for thrombosis and cardiovascular events.

8. Liver Dysfunction

- **Mechanism**: As PAI-1 is synthesized in the liver, any impairment of liver function, such as cirrhosis, fatty liver disease, or hepatitis, can alter PAI-1 production. Liver dysfunction can either increase or decrease PAI-1, depending on the stage and extent of liver damage.

9. Hypoxia

- **Mechanism**: Low oxygen conditions (hypoxia) can stimulate the production of PAI-1. Hypoxia-inducible factor-1α (HIF-1α) can activate the PAI-1 gene, leading to increased levels during conditions such as obstructive sleep apnea and chronic lung disease.

10. Medications

- **Mechanism**: Certain medications, such as **glucocorticoids**, **hormone replacement therapy**, or **oral contraceptives**, can increase PAI-1 production, potentially raising cardiovascular risk. This is particularly concerning for individuals with existing metabolic or cardiovascular conditions.

What are the consequences of elevated PAI-1?

- **Thrombosis**: By inhibiting fibrinolysis, elevated PAI-1 increases the risk of clot formation.

- **Atherosclerosis**: Promotes plaque formation and stability, heightening the risk of cardiovascular events.

- **Impaired wound healing**: Reduced fibrinolytic activity delays tissue repair and may contribute to chronic wounds in certain conditions.

Can you just decrease the PAI-1 levels?

Well, yes you can. You can decrease **PAI-1 (plasminogen activator inhibitor-1)** levels, particularly targeting the underlying conditions that elevate it, such as inflammation, metabolic issues, and endothelial dysfunction.

1. Lifestyle Modifications

- **Diet and Weight Management**: Obesity and metabolic syndrome are strongly associated with elevated PAI-1 levels. Studies show that **weight loss** through diet and exercise can significantly reduce PAI-1 concentrations. Diets rich in anti-inflammatory foods, such as the **Mediterranean diet**, which includes high intake of fruits, vegetables, whole grains, and healthy fats, have been shown to reduce PAI-1 levels.

- **Exercise**: Regular physical activity has been demonstrated to lower PAI-1 levels, likely by improving endothelial function and reducing inflammation and insulin resistance.

2. Pharmacological Interventions

- **Metformin**: Used primarily for the treatment of type 2 diabetes, **metformin** has been shown to decrease PAI-1 levels by improving insulin sensitivity and reducing inflammatory cytokines that stimulate PAI-1 production.

- **ACE Inhibitors/ARBs**: **Angiotensin-converting enzyme inhibitors** (ACE inhibitors) and **angiotensin receptor blockers** (ARBs) are commonly used in treating hypertension and heart disease. They can reduce PAI-1 by improving endothelial function and reducing vascular inflammation. Both medications have been suggested to play a role in modulating the renin-angiotensin system, which can influence PAI-1 levels.

- **Fibrates**: These drugs are used to lower triglyceride levels and may reduce PAI-1 levels in patients with metabolic syndrome or diabetes.

- **Statins**: Cholesterol-lowering statins, such as **atorvastatin**, have been shown to decrease PAI-1 levels by reducing systemic inflammation and improving endothelial health.

- **Pioglitazone**: A medication from the **thiazolidinedione** class, used for type 2 diabetes, has been shown to reduce PAI-1 levels by improving insulin resistance and decreasing inflammation.

3. Nutritional Supplements

- **Omega-3 Fatty Acids**: Found in fish oil and flaxseed oil, **omega-3 fatty acids** have anti-inflammatory properties and can help lower PAI-1 levels. They are known to improve endothelial function and reduce inflammation.

- **Resveratrol**: This polyphenol, found in red wine and grapes, has been shown to have anti-inflammatory and endothelial-protective effects, which can reduce PAI-1 levels.

- **Vitamin D**: Deficiency in vitamin D is associated with higher PAI-1 levels, and supplementation can reduce its concentrations by reducing inflammation and improving metabolic health.

4. Other Therapies

- **Glucagon-Like Peptide-1 (GLP-1) Agonists**: These drugs, used to treat diabetes, improve insulin sensitivity and reduce inflammation, which can help decrease PAI-1 levels.

- **Anti-Inflammatory Agents**: **Corticosteroids** or **biologic agents** that reduce chronic inflammation (e.g., anti-IL-6 agents) might also help in reducing PAI-1 levels by controlling cytokine production.

References:

1. **Mann, K. G., & Lenting, P. J.** (2023). Physiology, Coagulation Pathways. In *StatPearls*. StatPearls Publishing. https://www.ncbi.nlm.nih.gov/books/NBK482253/

2. **Barmore, W., Bajwa, T., & Burns, B.** (2023). Biochemistry, Clotting Factors. In *StatPearls*. StatPearls Publishing. https://www.ncbi.nlm.nih.gov/books/NBK507896/

3. Violi F, Harenberg J, Pignatelli P, Cammisotto V. COVID-19 and Long-COVID Thrombosis: From Clinical and Basic Science to Therapeutics. Thromb Haemost. 2024 Apr;124(4):286-296. doi: 10.1055/s-0043-1776713. Epub 2023 Nov 15. PMID: 37967846.

4. Taquet, M., Skorniewska, Z., Hampshire, A. *et al.* Acute blood biomarker profiles predict cognitive deficits 6 and 12 months after COVID-19 hospitalization. *Nat Med* **29**, 2498–2508 (2023). https://doi.org/10.1038/s41591-023-02525-y

5. Achleitner, M., Steenblock, C., Dänhardt, J. *et al.* Clinical improvement of Long-COVID is associated with reduction in autoantibodies, lipids, and inflammation following therapeutic apheresis. *Mol Psychiatry* **28**, 2872–2877 (2023). https://doi.org/10.1038/s41380-023-02084-1

6. Pretorius, E., Vlok, M., Venter, C., et al. (2021). Persistent clotting protein pathology in Long COVID/Post-Acute Sequelae of COVID-19 (PASC) is accompanied by increased levels of antiplasmin. *Cardiovascular Diabetology,* 20(1), 172. https://doi.org/10.1186/s12933-021-01359-7

7. Pretorius, E., Venter, C., Laubscher, G.J., et al. (2022). Persistent microclotting and platelet pathology in Long COVID/Post-Acute

Sequelae of COVID-19 (PASC): evidence of thrombotic endothelialitis and hyperactivated platelets. *Seminars in Thrombosis and Hemostasis*, 48(8), 859-868. https://doi.org/10.1055/a-1850-8478

8. Grobler, C., Maphumulo, S.C., Grobbelaar, L.M., et al. (2021). COVID-19: The Rollercoaster of Fibrin(ogen), D-dimer, von Willebrand Factor, P-Selectin and their Roles in Microthrombi Formation. *Cardiovascular Research*, 116(11), 2680-2692. https://doi.org/10.1093/cvr/cvaa282

9. Kell, D.B., Laubscher, G.J., & Pretorius, E. (2022). A central role for amyloid fibrin microclots in long COVID/PASC: origins and therapeutic implications. *Biochemical Journal*, 479(4), 537-559. https://doi.org/10.1042/BCJ20210792

10. von Meijenfeldt, F.A., Havervall, S., Adelmeijer, J., et al. (2022). Sustained prothrombotic changes in COVID-19 patients 4 months after hospital discharge. *Blood Advances*, 5(3), 756-761. https://doi.org/10.1182/bloodadvances.2020003992

11. Levi, M., Thachil, J., Iba, T., & Levy, J.H. (2021). Coagulation abnormalities and thrombosis in patients with COVID-19. *The Lancet Haematology*, 7(6), e438-e440. https://doi.org/10.1016/S2352-3026(20)30145-9

12. Platt, O. S., Thorington, B. D., Brambilla, D. J., et al. (1991). Pain in sickle cell disease: Rates and risk factors. *The New England Journal of Medicine*, 325(1), 11-16. https://doi.org/10.1056/NEJM199107043250103

13. Declerck, P. J., & Gils, A. (2013). Three decades of research on plasminogen activator inhibitor-1: a multifaceted serpin. *Seminars in Thrombosis and Hemostasis*, 39(4), 356–364. https://doi.org/10.1055/s-0033-1334489

14. Jadhav SB, Shah N, Rathi A, Rathi V, Rathi A. Serratiopeptidase: Insights into the therapeutic applications. Biotechnol Rep (Amst).

2020 Oct 17;28:e00544. doi: 10.1016/j.btre.2020.e00544. PMID: 33134103; PMCID: PMC7585045.

15. Sharma C, Jha NK, Meeran MFN, Patil CR, Goyal SN, Ojha S. Serratiopeptidase, A Serine Protease Anti-Inflammatory, Fibrinolytic, and Mucolytic Drug, Can Be a Useful Adjuvant for Management in COVID-19. Front Pharmacol. 2021 Jun 24;12:603997. doi: 10.3389/fphar.2021.603997. PMID: 34248612; PMCID: PMC8265778.

16. Kurosawa Y, Nirengi S, Homma T, Esaki K, Ohta M, Clark JF, Hamaoka T. A single-dose of oral nattokinase potentiates thrombolysis and anti-coagulation profiles. Sci Rep. 2015 Jun 25;5:11601. doi: 10.1038/srep11601. PMID: 26109079; PMCID: PMC4479826.

17. Hsia, C.-H., Shen, M.-C., Lin, J.-S., Wen, Y.-K., Hwang, K.-L., Cham, T.-M., & Yang, N.-C. (2009). Nattokinase decreases plasma levels of fibrinogen, factor VII, and factor VIII in human subjects. *Nutrition Research, 29*(3), 190-196. https://doi.org/10.1016/j.nutres.2009.01.009

18. Altaf, F., Wu, S., & Kasim, V. (2021). Role of Fibrinolytic Enzymes in Anti-Thrombosis Therapy. *Frontiers in Molecular Biosciences, 8*. https://doi.org/10.3389/fmolb.2021.680397

19. Felton GE. Fibrinolytic and antithrombotic action of bromelain may eliminate thrombosis in heart patients. Med Hypotheses. 1980 Nov;6(11):1123-33. doi: 10.1016/0306-9877(80)90134-6. PMID: 6256612

Antioxidant Supplements

Let us get more into the weeds with herbal and plant-derived supplements. These supplements are primarily antioxidants and will reduce oxidative stress, which helps with **mitochondrial dysfunction**. Supplements mostly come from seeds, beans, plants, fruit, flowers, bark, nuts, tea leaves, roots. While I encourage you to get these from eating, getting the required daily amounts from food alone is difficult. Pretty much anything alive will have internal antioxidants. These can be just as good as any pharmaceutical-grade medication.

All plants contain bioactive compounds like alkaloids, flavonoids, terpenoids, and polyphenols, which can exert various therapeutic effects. The effects of these compounds function together and often enhance the efficacy, especially when combined.

> *The biggest producer of oxidants in your body is your own mitochondria. Sure, we can also get a healthy dose of extra oxidants from ozone, smoking, cured meats, fatty diets, radiation, and UV rays. My advice is, don't help. Your body has enough to deal with on its own.*

What is the point of antioxidants anyway?

Because antioxidants are just strong reduction agents, their job is to neutralize highly oxidative compounds that have the potential to damage DNA, causing DNA strand breaks and mutations. Oxidative stress occurs due to an imbalance between *Reactive Oxygen Species* (ROS) production in your mitochondria and the cell's ability to neutralize and repair the resulting damage. We want to remove these reactive and oxidative molecules before they can damage our organs.

What is oxidation and reduction?

It can get very confusing, so let's break it down: There are multiple ways to look at oxidants and reducing agents.

- It is always a **give** and **take**.
    - When reducing agents give up electrons to oxidants, they become oxidized themselves while reducing the oxidant.
    - Likewise, when oxidizing agents steal electrons, they become reduced themselves while oxidizing the reductant.
- An **oxidant** has a strong desire for electrons. **Oxidants** are **greedy** and **selfish** for electrons. **Oxidants steal electrons.**
- A **reductant** has extra electrons to give up and prefers to donate its electrons. **Reductants** are **generous** with their electrons and give them up without any fuss.

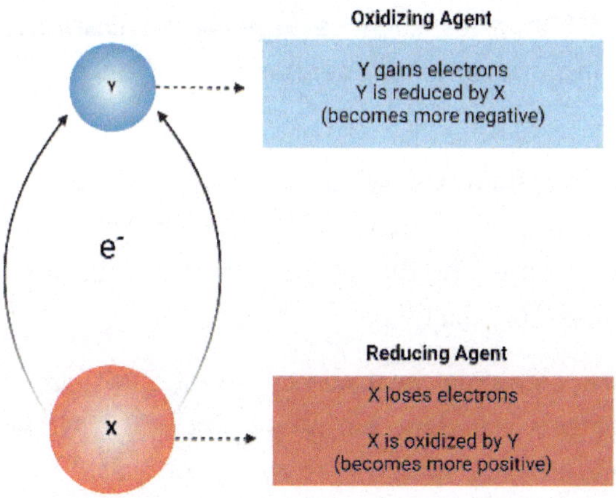

Antioxidants are nothing more than **potent reduction agents**. They have a tremendous capacity to give up their electrons to neutralize floating oxidants. Molecules can be labeled **strong reducers or weak reducers**. The stronger the reduction power, the easier it is for it to give up its electrons.

How do antioxidants work?

- **Reduce oxidative damage:** By scavenging ROS, antioxidants help protect cells and tissues from oxidative damage.
    - **Our built in "The Big Three" Antioxidant Enzymes**
        - **Superoxide Dismutase (SOD):** Converts superoxide into hydrogen peroxide.
        - **Catalase:** Converts hydrogen peroxide into water and oxygen.
        - **Glutathione Peroxidase:** Reduces hydrogen peroxide and organic hydroperoxides.
    - **Non-Enzymatic Antioxidants**
        - **Glutathione:** A tripeptide that directly scavenges ROS.
- **Upregulate antioxidant enzymes:** Polyphenols can stimulate the activity of enzymes such as **Superoxide Dismutase (SOD)** and **glutathione peroxidase**, enhancing the body's antioxidant capacity.
- **Inhibit pro-inflammatory cytokines:** Compounds like quercetin and resveratrol can downregulate the production of inflammatory cytokines (these are the proteins responsible for inflammation) such as IL-6, TNF-α, and IL-1β.
- **Modulate signaling pathways:** Polyphenols can influence key inflammatory signaling pathways, including **NF-κB** and **MAPK**, thereby reducing inflammatory responses. These signaling pathways work directly on the genes in the DNA inside the nucleus to either produce more or less of the inflammatory proteins.

Oxidative Stress Reduction (Antioxidant Therapy)

It is the broadest category. Antioxidants can help mitigate oxidative stress and protect mitochondria from damage. Oxidative stress occurs due to anything that adds oxidative potential to your cells.

How does an oxidant cause damage to a cell?

External strong oxidants such as ozone (O_3) and hydrogen peroxide (H_2O_2) and internally formed oxidants steal electrons from protein, fat, and DNA. These actions can deform proteins and damage DNA. It alters the molecule's shape and function. It can destabilize cell membranes, break DNA strands, or cause mutations. If enough mitochondria are damaged, the cell may die.

Ozone is a gas at room temperature and unstable because it has 3 oxygen molecules stuck together, O_3. It is unstable and wants to throw off the extra oxygen singlet so that a more stable O_2 can occur. It is a decomposition reaction and it is unstable. That single oxygen molecule is also an oxidant. You get two oxidants in one! Isn't that special? Isn't ozone awesome?

When ozone is infused into the bloodstream, it quickly combines with water in your blood to form hydrogen peroxide, also an oxidant. This is the primary reason why I do not recommend ozone-type treatments.

Antioxidant supplements come in various forms and include a range of vitamins, minerals, and other compounds that help protect the body from oxidative stress. Here are some commonly available antioxidant supplements. It is essential to know that some antioxidants can act as pro-oxidants and become toxic if taken excessively. More is not always better. While not necessarily recommended, those marked with an * below can also become pro-oxidants if taken excessively. Prooxidants would do the opposite of what we want and become oxidants. Don't be scared to take these; just don't overdo it.

- Chromium*
- Cobalt*
- Vanadium*
- Nickel*
- Manganese*
- Iron*
- Copper *
- Selenium *
- Zinc *
- Magnesium

Vitamins

1. Vitamin C (Ascorbic Acid) *
2. Vitamin E (Tocopherol)
3. Vitamin A (Beta-Carotene)
4. Vitamin D
5. Vitamin K

Antioxidants – A to Z

+ increases the risk of bleeding.

- Acai Berry
- Aloe Vera
- Alpha-Lipoic Acid (ALA)
- Anthocyanins (found in berries)
- Apigenin
- Arginine
- Ashwagandha

- Astaxanthin
- Bilberry
- Blueberry Extract
- Bromelain +
- Carnitine
- Catechins (found in green tea)
- Chlorella (algae that grow in freshwater. It is sometimes called seaweed)
- **Chlorophyll** (found in green leafy vegetables)
- Coenzyme Q10 (CoQ10)
- Cranberry Extract+
- Curcumin/turmeric
- Cysteine
- Elderberry
- Epicatechin (cocoa)
- Feverfew (flower)
- Fisetin
- **Fulvic acid** and **humic acid** are organic compounds found in soil, peat, coal, and bodies of water. They are both products of the decomposition of organic matter.
- Garlic+
- Ginger+
- Ginkgo Biloba+
- Ginseng
- **Glucosinolates** (found in *cruciferous* vegetables like broccoli)
- Glutathione

- Goji Berry
- Grape Seed Extract+
- Green Tea Extract (EGCG)+
- Hesperidin
- Histidine
- Holy Basil (Tulsi) is different from ordinary basil.
- Kaempferol
- Lutein
- Luteolin
- Lycopene
- Lumbrokinase +
- Lysine
- Mangosteen (fruit) +
- Medium chain fatty acids (MCFA)
- Melatonin
- Methionine
- Methylene blue – careful with renal failure, G6PD deficiency, on SSRIs, cyproheptadine, MAO inhibitors
- N-acetylcysteine (NAC)
- Nattokinase +
- Omega 3- fatty acids/fish oils
- Palmitoylethanolamide (PEA)
- Pycnogenol (pine bark extract)
- Quercetin +
- Resveratrol
- Rhodiola Rosea (golden root)

- Rutin
- Silymarin (found in milk thistle)
- Spirulina (blue-green algae)
- sulforaphane (Broccoli, Bok choy, cabbage)
- Taurine
- Theaflavin (black tea)
- Tryptophan
- Turmeric (Curcumin)+
- Tyrosine
- Uric acid
- Zeaxanthin

There are hundreds more. The point is, when selecting antioxidants, it is crucial to choose from diverse categories. Ones in the same categories tend to have the same characteristics. By selecting one from each category, you can ensure that you diversify their impact.

Flow chart for polyphenols

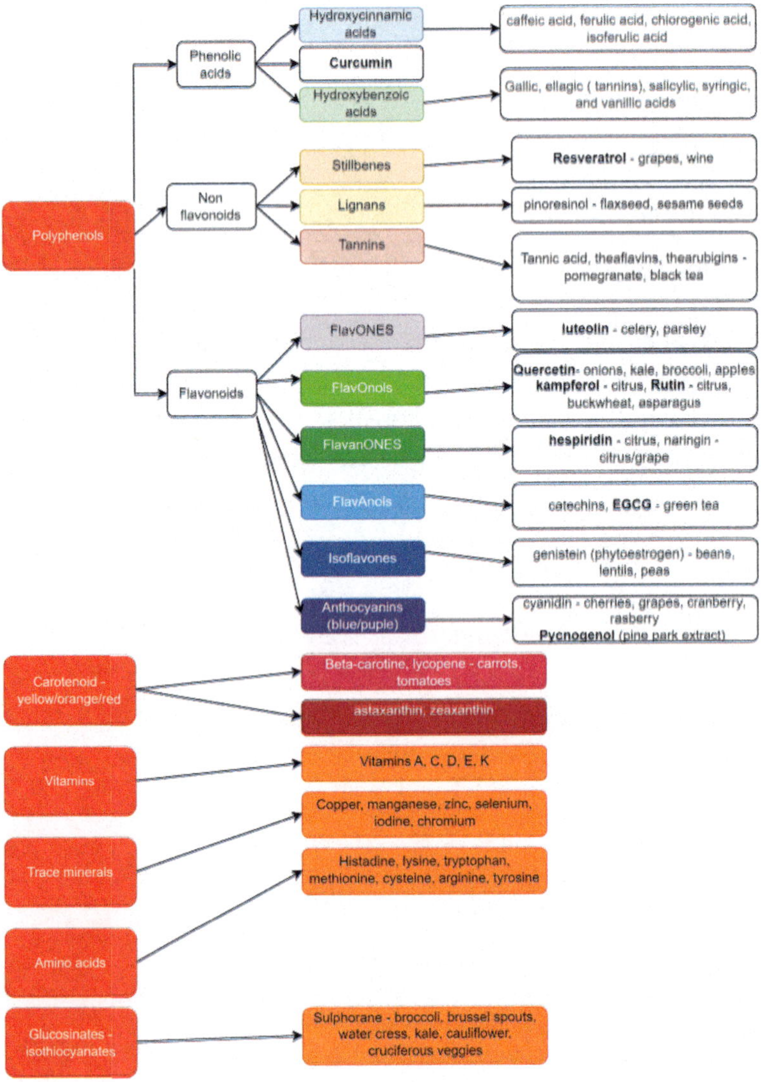
Polyphenols
Phenolic acids
Hydroxycinnamic acids
caffeic acid, ferulic acid, chlorogenic acid, isoferulic acid
Curcumin
Hydroxybenzoic acids
Gallic, ellagic (tannins), salicylic, syringic, and vanillic acids
Non flavonoids
Stillbenes
Resveratrol - grapes, wine
Lignans
pinoresinol - flaxseed, sesame seeds
Tannins
Tannic acid, theaflavins, thearubigins - pomegranate, black tea
Flavonoids
FlavONES
luteolin - celery, parsley
FlavOnols
Quercetin- onions, kale, broccoli, apples kampferol - citrus, Rutin - citrus, buckwheat, asparagus
FlavanONES
hespiridin - citrus, naringin - citrus/grape
FlavAnols
catechins, EGCG - green tea
Isoflavones
genistein (phytoestrogen) - beans, lentils, peas
Anthocyanins (blue/puple)
cyanidin - cherries, grapes, cranberry, rasberry Pycnogenol (pine park extract)
Carotenoid - yellow/orange/red
Beta-carotine, lycopene - carrots, tomatoes
astaxanthin, zeaxanthin
Vitamins
Vitamins A, C, D, E, K
Trace minerals
Copper, manganese, zinc, selenium, iodine, chromium
Amino acids
Histadine, lysine, tryptophan, methionine, cysteine, arginine, tyrosine
Glucosinates - isothiocyanates
Sulphorane - broccoli, brussel spouts, water cress, kale, cauliflower, cruciferous veggies

References:

2. Burton GJ, Jauniaux E. Oxidative stress. Best Pract Res Clin Obstet Gynaecol. 2011 Jun;25(3):287-99. DOI:

10.1016/j.bpobgyn.2010.10.016. Epub 2010 Dec 3. PMID: 21130690; PMCID: PMC3101336.

3. Sies, H. Oxidative Stress: Concept and Some Practical Aspects. *Antioxidants* **2020**, *9*, 852.

https://DOI.org/10.3390/antiox9090852

4. Abeyrathne EDNS, Nam K, Huang X, Ahn DU. Plant- and Animal-Based Antioxidants' Structure, Efficacy, Mechanisms, and Applications: A Review. Antioxidants (Basel). 2022 May 23;11(5):1025. DOI: 10.3390/antiox11051025. PMID: 35624889; PMCID: PMC9137533.

5. Di Gioia F, Tzortzakis N, Rouphael Y, Kyriacou MC, Sampaio SL, Ferreira ICFR, Petropoulos SA. Grown to be Blue-Antioxidant Properties and Health Effects of Colored Vegetables. Part II: Leafy, Fruit, and Other Vegetables. Antioxidants (Basel). 2020 Jan 23;9(2):97. DOI:

10.3390/antiox9020097. PMID: 31979214; PMCID:

PMC7070715.

6. Khoo HE, Azlan A, Tang ST, Lim SM. Anthocyanidins and anthocyanins: colored pigments as food, pharmaceutical ingredients, and the potential health benefits. Food Nutr Res. 2017 Aug 13;61(1):1361779. DOI:

10.1080/16546628.2017.1361779. PMID: 28970777;

PMCID: PMC5613902.

7. Cosme F, Pinto T, Aires A, Morais MC, Bacelar E, Anjos R, Ferreira-Cardoso J, Oliveira I, Vilela A, Gonçalves B. Red Fruits Composition and Their Health Benefits-A Review. Foods. 2022 Feb 23;11(5):644. DOI: 10.3390/foods11050644. PMID: 35267278; PMCID: PMC8909293.

8. Nobile V, Pisati M, Cestone E, Insolia V, Zaccaria V, Malfa GA. Antioxidant Efficacy of a Standardized Red Orange (*Citrus sinensis* (L.) Osbeck) Extract in Elderly Subjects: A Randomized, Double Blind,

Controlled Study. Nutrients. 2022 Oct 11;14(20):4235. DOI: 10.3390/nu14204235. PMID: 36296919; PMCID: PMC9611767.

9. Red Fruits: Extraction of Antioxidants, Phenolic Content, and Radical Scavenging Determination: A Review. *Antioxidants*. 2017;6(1):7. DOI:10.3390/antiox6010007.

10. Cömert ED, Mogol BA, Gökmen V. Relationship between color and antioxidant capacity of fruits and vegetables. Curr Res Food Sci. 2019 Nov 21;2:1-10. DOI:

10.1016/j.crfs.2019.11.001. PMID: 32914105; PMCID: PMC7473347.

11. Forman, H.J., Zhang, H. Targeting oxidative stress in disease: promise and limitations of antioxidant therapy. *Nat Rev Drug Discov* **20**, 689–709 (2021). https://DOI.org/10.1038/s41573-021-00233-1

12. https://www.medicalnewstoday.com/articles/324863

13. García-Sánchez, A., Miranda-Díaz, A. G., & Cardona-Muñoz, E. G. (2020). The role of oxidative stress in physiopathology and pharmacological treatment with pro- and antioxidant properties in chronic diseases. *Oxidative Medicine and Cellular Longevity*. https://DOI.org/10.1155/2020/2082145

14. Abdelazim, A. M., & Abomughaid, M. M. (2024). Oxidative stress: an overview of past research and future insights. *All Life*, *17*(1). https://DOI.org/10.1080/26895293.2024.2316092

15. Chaudhary P, Janmeda P, Docea AO, et al. Oxidative stress, free radicals and antioxidants: potential crosstalk in the pathophysiology of human diseases. *Front Chem*. 2023; 11:1158198. DOI:10.3389/fchem.2023.1158198.

What is Mitochondrial Dysfunction?

Let's talk about mitochondria for a moment. They are tiny organelles inside cells. Organelles are like mini factories inside your cells. The mitochondrial number in each cell depends on what the organ does and how much energy the cells of the organ require. Some organs are very energy intensive, for instance, to move ions against their gradient, produce substances, contracting a muscle, or move around.

Mitochondria are factories inside cells responsible for producing *Adenosine Triphosphate* (ATP), the primary energy currency of the cell, through oxidative phosphorylation. They also regulate cellular metabolism, apoptosis (cell death), and Reactive Oxygen Species (ROS) production.

Some of our most energy-intensive organs are the brain, nerves, heart, muscles, liver, kidneys, pancreas, and gastrointestinal tract. It is not a surprise that Long COVID happens to target these organs. When COVID infects cells, these are more likely to have problems later on due to mitochondrial damage.

The COVID-19 virus directly damages mitochondria. Mitochondrial dysfunction has emerged as a potential underlying factor in Long COVID. Furthermore, cells and mitochondria produce abnormal proteins that impair the electron transport chain and interfere with energy production.

Mitochondrial dysfunction occurs when these factories fail to produce adequate energy, often due to impaired oxidative phosphorylation, increased ROS production, or mitochondrial DNA (mtDNA) damage. This dysfunction can lead to cellular energy deficits, increased oxidative stress, and subsequent tissue and organ damage. ROS can damage our DNA by causing mutations and DNA strand breaks. Lactic acid may build up. As I said earlier, our bodies do not need your help with extra oxidants.

Mitochondrial damage and dysfunction are a **secondary cause**. You were not born with bad mitochondria; they were damaged by disease. Not every mitochondrion in every organ would be affected. This scenario would be individual and unique to each person. Depending on which organs were involved determines the symptoms.

Mechanisms

- **Oxidative Stress and Inflammation** - During acute COVID-19, an elevated immune response can lead to excessive production of ROS, resulting in oxidative stress. Consequently, chronic inflammation and oxidative stress can damage mitochondrial membranes, proteins, and DNA, impairing their function and contributing to persistent symptoms in Long COVID.

- **Energy Deficits** - Mitochondrial dysfunction reduces ATP production, causing energy deficits in various tissues. It can manifest as fatigue, muscle weakness, and exercise intolerance, which Long COVID patients commonly report.

- **Abnormal Protein Interference –** abnormal protein accumulation inside mitochondria can disrupt the typical electron transport chain and ATP production. Moreover, it appears to be associated with the WASF3 protein.

References:

- Zong, Y., Li, H., Liao, P. *et al.* Mitochondrial dysfunction: mechanisms and advances in therapy. *Sig Transduct Target Ther* 9, 124 (2024). https://doi.org/10.1038/s41392-024-01839-8

- Giulivi, C., Zhang, K. & Arakawa, H. Recent advances and new perspectives in mitochondrial dysfunction. *Sci Rep* **13**, 7977 (2023). https://doi.org/10.1038/s41598-023-34624-8

- Molnar, T., Lehoczki, A., Fekete, M. *et al.* Mitochondrial dysfunction in long COVID: mechanisms, consequences, and potential therapeutic approaches. *GeroScience* **46**, 5267–5286 (2024). https://doi.org/10.1007/s11357-024-01165-5

- Appelman, B., Charlton, B.T., Goulding, R.P. *et al.* Muscle abnormalities worsen after post-exertional malaise in long COVID. *Nat Commun* **15**, 17 (2024). https://doi.org/10.1038/s41467-023-44432-3

- Kunwadee, N., Chatatikun, M., Sirirat, S., Kotepui, M., Rahni, H., Bunluepuech, K., Noothong, C., Tedasen, A., Klangbud, W. K., Imai, M., Kawakami, F., Kubo, M., Kitagawa, Y., Ichikawa, H., Kanekura, T., Sukati, S., Somsak, V., Lunla, U., Ichikawa, T., Nissapatorn, V., Tangpong, J., Indo, H. P., & Majima, H. J. (2023). Mitochondrial oxidative stress, mitochondrial ROS storms in long COVID pathogenesis. *Frontiers in Immunology, 14.* https://doi.org/10.3389/fimmu.2023.1275001

- Wang, P., Ma, J., Kim, Y.-C., & Hwang, P. M. (2023). WASF3 disrupts mitochondrial respiration and may mediate exercise intolerance in myalgic encephalomyelitis/chronic fatigue syndrome. *Proceedings of the National Academy of Sciences*, 120(34), e23027381. https://doi.org/10.1073/pnas.2302738120

- Guarnieri, J. W., Dybas, J. M., & Wallace, D. C., et al. (2023). Core mitochondrial genes are down-regulated during SARS-CoV-2 infection of rodent and human hosts. Science Translational Medicine, 15(708), eabq1533. https://doi.org/10.1126/scitranslmed.abq1533

Apoptosis, Autophagy, Mitophagy, and Cellular Damage

Mitochondria play a crucial role in regulating apoptosis or programmed cell death. Dysfunctional mitochondria can trigger inappropriate apoptosis, leading to tissue damage and multi-system involvement in Long COVID. Because mitochondria need to signal for cell death, dysfunctional mitochondria may prevent not only a cell from functioning correctly but also from dying when it needs to.

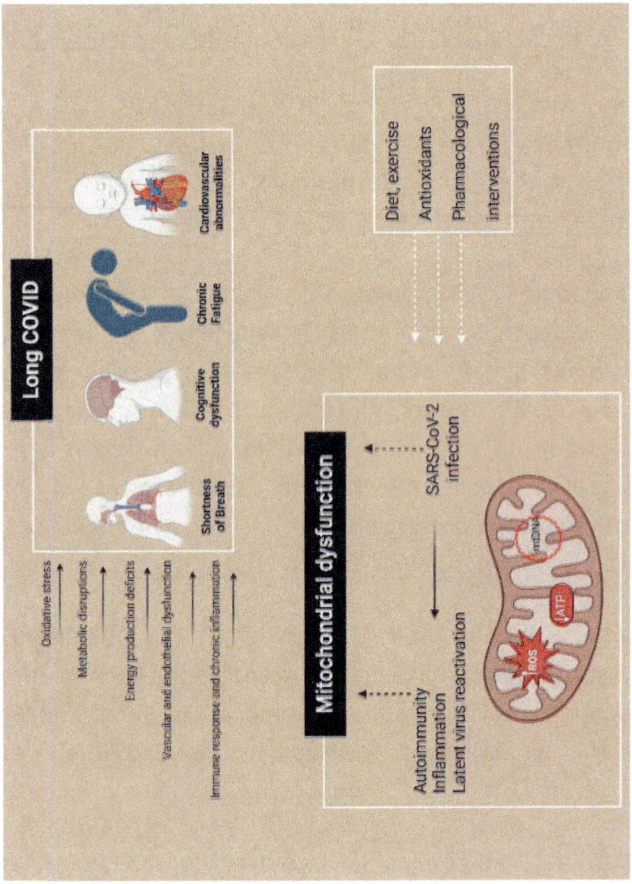

Apoptosis lets us destroy and remove damaged cells that are not doing anything useful. These damaged cells cannot multiple/divide or die off. This is because healthy mitochondria are required for cell to die off in a programmed way. They use energy and create a lot of Reactive Oxidative Species (ROS), also known as free radicals, but don't do anything useful.

Fun fact: mitochondria control when a cell can die thru apoptosis/autophagy/mitophagy. If there is no signal, then there is no cell death.

Step 2 is short. We want to get in, kill the enemies, and get out. If this is ongoing, you will begin to kill off healthy mitochondria, which will be counterproductive. There is more than one type of signal that is used to start apoptosis. We want apoptosis instead of necrosis because the former is non-inflammatory.

Metformin can increase lactic acid levels by slowing down the Krebs cycle, which may seem counterintuitive since the Krebs cycle generates ATP, but it allows the mitochondria to rest.

There are several signals that can start the apoptosis process

- Intermittent fasting
- **Apigenin** – induces apoptosis by increasing the expression of **pro-apoptotic proteins** (e.g., Bax) and decreases the levels of **anti-apoptotic proteins** (e.g., Bcl-2). Note, apigenin can increase ROS production.
- **mTOR inhibitor: Rapamycin,** lipoic acid, resveratrol, **Urolithin A**
- <u>Sirt1 activation:</u> **ferulic acid**, **melatonin**, **urolithin A (skeletal muscles)**, **resveratrol**, **metformin** (short term only)
    - Liver, skeletal muscles, pancreas, brain
- <u>AMPK activation:</u> **metformin** and **berberine**
    - It is constructive for liver and white blood cell function
- <u>Nrf2 activation:</u> **lipoic acid**, broccoli sprout extract
- <u>PPARα activation:</u> **astaxanthin**

References:

- Kim TW, Lee HG. Apigenin Induces Autophagy and Cell Death by Targeting EZH2 under Hypoxia Conditions in Gastric Cancer Cells. Int J Mol Sci. 2021 Dec 15;22(24):13455. doi: 10.3390/ijms222413455. PMID: 34948250; PMCID: PMC8706813.

- Halma, M. T. J., Marik, P. E., & Saleeby, Y. M. (2024). Exploring autophagy in treating SARS-CoV-2 spike protein-related pathology. *Endocrine and Metabolic Science, 14,* 100163. https://doi.org/10.1016/j.endmts.2024.100163

- Husain A, Byrareddy SN. Rapamycin as a potential repurpose drug candidate for the treatment of COVID-19. Chem Biol Interact. 2020 Nov 1;331:109282. doi: 10.1016/j.cbi.2020.109282. Epub 2020 Oct 6. PMID: 33031791; PMCID: PMC7536130.

- Karp, A. (2021). Rapamycin and Metformin in Treating COVID-19. *The Science Journal of the Lander College of Arts and Sciences, 14*(2), 43-51.

- Wu, J., Bai, Y., Wang, Y., & Ma, J. (2021). Melatonin and regulation of autophagy: Mechanisms and therapeutic implications. *Pharmacological Research, 163,* 105279. https://doi.org/10.1016/j.phrs.2020.105279

- Boga, J. A., Caballero, B., Potes, Y., Perez-Martinez, Z., Reiter, R. J., Vega-Naredo, I., & Coto-Montes, A. (2018). Therapeutic potential of melatonin related to its role as an autophagy regulator: A review. *Journal of Pineal Research*. https://doi.org/10.1111/jpi.12534

- Jayatunga DPW, Hone E, Khaira H, Lunelli T, Singh H, Guillemin GJ, Fernando B, Garg ML, Verdile G, Martins RN. Therapeutic Potential of Mitophagy-Inducing Microflora Metabolite, Urolithin A for Alzheimer's Disease. Nutrients. 2021 Oct 23;13(11):3744. doi: 10.3390/nu13113744. PMID: 34836000; PMCID: PMC8617978.

- Andreux, P.A., Blanco-Bose, W., Ryu, D. *et al.* The mitophagy activator urolithin A is safe and induces a molecular signature of improved mitochondrial and cellular health in humans. *Nat Metab* **1**, 595–603 (2019). https://doi.org/10.1038/s42255-019-0073-4

- Faitg J, D'Amico D, Rinsch C, Singh A. Mitophagy Activation by Urolithin A to Target Muscle Aging. Calcif Tissue Int. 2024 Jan;114(1):53-59. doi: 10.1007/s00223-023-01145-5. Epub 2023 Nov 5. PMID: 37925671; PMCID: PMC10791945.

- Park, D., Jeong, H., Lee, M. *et al.* Resveratrol induces autophagy by directly inhibiting mTOR through ATP competition. *Sci Rep* **6**, 21772 (2016). https://doi.org/10.1038/srep21772

- Li J, Fan Y, Zhang Y, Liu Y, Yu Y, Ma M. Resveratrol Induces Autophagy and Apoptosis in Non-Small-Cell Lung Cancer Cells by Activating the NGFR-AMPK-mTOR Pathway. Nutrients. 2022 Jun 10;14(12):2413. doi: 10.3390/nu14122413. PMID: 35745143; PMCID: PMC9228598.

- Narasimman Gurusamy, Istvan Lekli, Subhendu Mukherjee, Diptarka Ray, Md. Kaimul Ahsan, Mihaela Gherghiceanu, Lawrence M. Popescu, Dipak K. Das, Cardioprotection by resveratrol: a novel mechanism via autophagy involving the mTORC2 pathway, *Cardiovascular Research*, Volume 86, Issue 1, 1 April 2010, Pages 103–112, https://doi.org/10.1093/cvr/cvp384

- de Marañón AM, Díaz-Pozo P, Canet F, Díaz-Morales N, Abad-Jiménez Z, López-Domènech S, Vezza T, Apostolova N, Morillas C, Rocha M, Víctor VM. Metformin modulates mitochondrial function and mitophagy in peripheral blood mononuclear cells from type 2 diabetic patients. Redox Biol. 2022 Jul;53:102342. doi: 10.1016/j.redox.2022.102342. Epub 2022 May 17. PMID: 35605453; PMCID: PMC9124713.

- Foretz, M., Guigas, B. & Viollet, B. Metformin: update on mechanisms of action and repurposing potential. *Nat Rev Endocrinol* **19**, 460–476 (2023). https://doi.org/10.1038/s41574-023-00833-4

- Um JH, Lee KM, Kim YY, Lee DY, Kim E, Kim DH, Yun J. Berberine Induces Mitophagy through Adenosine Monophosphate-Activated Protein Kinase and Ameliorates Mitochondrial Dysfunction in

PINK1 Knockout Mouse Embryonic Fibroblasts. Int J Mol Sci. 2023 Dec 22;25(1):219. doi: 10.3390/ijms25010219. PMID: 38203389; PMCID: PMC10779002.

- Tang, L., Zhang, Y., Jobson, H. E., Li, J., Stephenson, K. K., Wade, K. L., & Fahey, J. W. (2006). Potent activation of mitochondria-mediated apoptosis and arrest in S and M phases of cancer cells by a broccoli sprout extract. *Molecular Cancer Therapeutics, 5*(4), 935–944. https://doi.org/10.1158/1535-7163.MCT-05-0476

- Nishida Y, Nawaz A, Hecht K, Tobe K. Astaxanthin as a Novel Mitochondrial Regulator: A New Aspect of Carotenoids, beyond Antioxidants. Nutrients. 2021 Dec 27;14(1):107. doi: 10.3390/nu14010107. PMID: 35010981; PMCID: PMC8746862.

- Peng, P., Zhang, X., Qi, T., Cheng, H., Kong, Q., Liu, L., Cao, X., & Ding, Z. (2020). Alpha-lipoic acid inhibits lung cancer growth via mTOR-mediated autophagy inhibition. *FEBS Open Bio, 10*(5), 837–844. https://doi.org/10.1002/2211-5463.12820

Intermittent Fasting

Intermittent fasting is an eating pattern where you cycle between periods of eating and fasting. It is different from just fasting, which is basically starvation. One of the key benefits of intermittent fasting is its potential to trigger **autophagy**, a natural process where your body cleans out damaged cells and regenerates new, healthier ones.

During fasting, when your body has depleted its glucose stores and insulin levels drop, cells initiate **autophagy**. This process involves breaking down old or damaged proteins and organelles to maintain cellular health. **Autophagy** plays a crucial role in reducing inflammation, improving metabolic function, and potentially slowing the aging process. It has also been studied for its role in preventing or managing diseases like cancer, neurodegenerative disorders, and heart disease.

How intermittent fasting triggers autophagy

- Fasting leads to nutrient deprivation, which prompts cells to begin cleaning themselves.
- By eliminating damaged parts, cells increase their efficiency and reduce the risk of age-related diseases.
- Research shows that fasting for 16-24 hours can increase autophagy activity, although the exact timing varies among individuals.

Benefits of autophagy through intermittent fasting

- **Cellular rejuvenation**: Helps repair and regenerate cells.
- **Disease prevention**: May lower the risk of conditions like Alzheimer's, Parkinson's, and certain cancers by removing damaged cells.
- **Improved metabolic health**: Can help regulate blood sugar and insulin sensitivity.
- **Anti-aging effects**: Reducing cellular damage can slow down the aging process.

How do you do intermittent fasting safely?

involves several key steps to ensure you get the benefits without harming your health:

1. How to Start?

If you're new to fasting, start with a mild schedule like the **12:12 method** (12 hours of fasting, 12 hours of eating) and gradually work your way up to more challenging patterns, such as the **16:8 method** (16 hours of fasting, 8 hours of eating). You can do it 3 days a week. It's not necessary to do intermittent fasting every day. You can use intermittent fasting as part of **Step 2** of my protocol.

2. Stay Hydrated

During fasting periods, make sure to drink plenty of water. You can also consume unsweetened tea, black coffee, or electrolyte drinks (without calories) to avoid dehydration. Anything without calories is fine.

3. Eat Nutrient-Dense Foods

During your eating windows, focus on whole, nutrient-rich foods like fruits, vegetables, lean proteins, whole grains, and healthy fats. This ensures your body gets essential nutrients to support energy levels and overall health.

4. Listen to Your Body

If you feel dizzy, overly fatigued, or unwell while fasting, it's essential to stop and eat. Fasting should not lead to extreme discomfort. If needed, consult a healthcare provider before continuing.

5. Avoid Overeating

When your eating window opens, avoid the temptation to binge or consume large amounts of unhealthy food. Overeating can cause digestive issues and negate the benefits of fasting.

6. Consult a Doctor Before Starting

It's crucial to consult with a healthcare provider before starting intermittent fasting, especially if you have underlying medical conditions like **diabetes, heart disease**, or are **pregnant** or **breastfeeding**. They can provide personalized guidance based on your health needs.

7. Monitor energy and nutrient intake

If intermittent fasting leads to reduced calorie intake, be mindful to avoid deficiencies in key nutrients like vitamins and minerals. Consider tracking your meals to ensure balanced nutrition.

References:

1. Patterson, R. E., & Sears, D. D. (2017). "Metabolic Effects of Intermittent Fasting." *Annual Review of Nutrition*. https://doi.org/10.1146/annurev-nutr-071816-064634

2. Anton, S. D., et al. (2018). "Flipping the Metabolic Switch: Understanding and Applying the Health Benefits of Fasting." *Obesity*. https://doi.org/10.1002/oby.22168

3. Longo, V. D., & Panda, S. (2016). "Fasting, Circadian Rhythms, and Time-Restricted Feeding in Healthy Lifespan." *Cell Metabolism*. https://doi.org/10.1016/j.cmet.2016.06.001

4. Madeo, F., Zimmermann, A., & Carmona-Gutierrez, D. (2015). "The connection between autophagy and longevity." *Nature Reviews Molecular Cell Biology*. https://doi.org/10.1038/nrm4025

5. Anton, S. D., Moehl, K., Donahoo, W. T., et al. (2018). "Flipping the Metabolic Switch: Understanding and Applying the Health Benefits of Fasting." *Obesity*. https://doi.org/10.1002/oby.22168

6. Levine, B., & Kroemer, G. (2019). "Biological Functions of Autophagy Genes: A Disease Perspective." *Cell*. https://doi.org/10.1016/j.cell.2019.10.037

Treating Mitochondrial Dysfunction

Mitochondrial dysfunction targets cells in organs that are energy or metabolism dependent. Some vital ones are nerves, brain, heart, liver, muscles, kidneys, and pancreas. The symptoms reflect dysfunction in these organs.

Mitochondria—often called the cell's powerhouse—is integral to energy production and cellular metabolism. Dysfunctional mitochondria can lead to a range of symptoms commonly observed in Long COVID:

- fatigue
- muscle weakness, muscle atrophy
- cognitive impairment
- visual and hearing problems
- heart, liver, and kidney disease
- thyroid dysfunction
- diabetes
- adrenal dysfunction
- autonomic nervous system dysfunction
- neurologic problems
- seizures

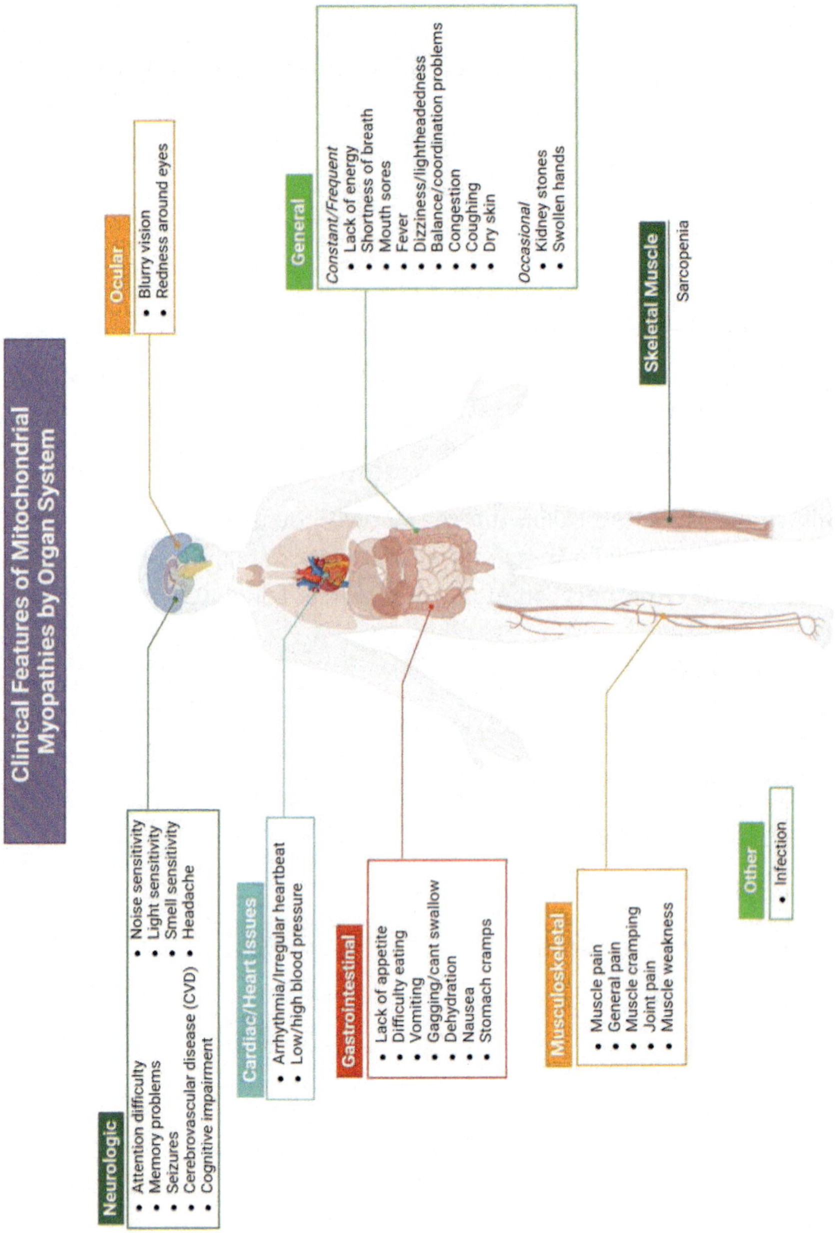

Clinical Features of Mitochondrial Myopathies by Organ System
Neurologic
• Attention difficulty
• Memory problems
• Seizures
• Cerebrovascular disease (CVD)
• Cognitive impairment
• Noise sensitivity
• Light sensitivity
• Smell sensitivity
• Headache
Ocular
• Blurry vision
• Redness around eyes
Cardiac/Heart Issues
• Arrhythmia/Irregular heartbeat
• Low/high blood pressure
General
Constant/Frequent
• Lack of energy
• Shortness of breath
• Mouth sores
• Fever
• Dizziness/lightheadedness
• Balance/coordination problems
• Congestion
• Coughing
• Dry skin
Occasional
• Kidney stones
• Swollen hands
Gastrointestinal
• Lack of appetite
• Difficulty eating
• Vomiting
• Gagging/cant swallow
• Dehydration
• Nausea
• Stomach cramps
Skeletal Muscle
Sarcopenia
Musculoskeletal
• Muscle pain
• General pain
• Muscle cramping
• Joint pain
• Muscle weakness
Other
• Infection

Yes, you read that right! It can cause involve several organs and cause very diverse symptoms. I typically examine muscle weakness, fatigue, brain fog, and shortness of breath.

Shortness of Breath

- The muscles between your ribs, intercostal muscles, and diaphragm are skeletal and can weaken due to mitochondrial dysfunction. It can make you feel short of breath.

- Another reason this might happen is a shortage of ATP production, which relies more and more on anaerobic metabolism despite having oxygen. This can occur due to increased oxidative stress, which reduces mitochondrial efficiency.

The 4 Treatment Steps

I will address how I treat mitochondrial dysfunction more in the book *The Complete Long COVID Handbook: Mitochondrial Dysfunction*. These 4-steps are given as follows:

1. Reduce oxidative stress
2. Remove damaged mitochondria (mitophagy)
3. Increase mitochondria numbers in healthy cells
4. Support mitochondrial metabolic mechanisms

Step 1: Reduce Oxidative Stress - Antioxidant Therapy

Step 1 continues throughout the treatment. Antioxidants are best for this; this treatment continues throughout the entire mitochondrial treatment set of steps. They can help reduce oxidative stress and protect mitochondria from damage.

Step 2: Autophagy and Mitophagy

Let's destroy and remove those cells that are not doing anything valuable. They use energy and create a lot of Reactive Oxidative Species (ROS), also known as free radicals, but don't do anything useful. Fun fact: mitochondria control when a cell can die. There is no signal, no death, and no division either. This step is short. We want to get in, kill the enemies, and get out. If this is ongoing, you will begin to kill off healthy mitochondria, which will be counterproductive.

Metformin can aggravate lactic acid levels by slowing down the Krebs cycle, which may seem counterintuitive since the Krebs cycle generates ATP, but it allows the mitochondria to rest. The signal is listed followed by supplements and medications that use it.

- Intermittent fasting
- **Apigenin** – induces apoptosis
- mTOR inhibition **– Rapamycin, Urolithin A**
- Sirt1 activation: ferulic acid, **melatonin**, **urolithin A (skeletal muscles)**, glucosamine, **resveratrol**, **metformin** (short term only)
  - Liver, skeletal muscles, pancreas, brain
- AMPK activation: **metformin** and **berberine**
  - It is constructive for liver and white blood cell function
- Nrf2 activation: **lipoic acid**, broccoli sprout extract
- PPARα activation: **astaxanthin**

Step 3: Mitochondrial Biogenesis

Certain compounds can promote mitochondrial biogenesis, forming new mitochondria either from scratch or from the fission of existing mitochondria. This step can continue till the end of treatment within 30-90 days.

- **PQQ (Pyrroloquinoline Quinone)** - a redox cofactor that promotes **mitochondrial biogenesis** and protects existing mitochondria from oxidative damage. Supplementing with PQQ can enhance cellular energy production and reduce fatigue.
- **Honokiol** (magnolia extract) – skeletal muscle and nerves; crosses blood-brain barrier. It has shown promise in Parkinson's and ALS.
- **Fisetin** – nerve focus.

- **Low dose naltrexone (LDN)**
- Creatine

Step 4: Make it easier to make energy – support

Proper nutrition is vital for maintaining mitochondrial health and function.

- **B Vitamins** - particularly B1 (thiamine), B2 (riboflavin), B3 (niacin), B5 (pantothenic acid), and B12 (cobalamin), are crucial for mitochondrial energy production. Ensuring adequate intake of these vitamins through diet or supplementation can support mitochondrial function.
- **Magnesium** is a cofactor for many enzymatic reactions in the mitochondria, including ATP synthesis. Supplementing with magnesium can improve mitochondrial function and reduce muscle fatigue.
- **L-Carnitine** - is involved in transporting fatty acids into mitochondria for energy production.
- **CoQ10** - a crucial component of the electron transport chain in mitochondria, playing a pivotal role in ATP production.
- **α-Lipoic Acid (ALA)** used together with **α-Ketoglutaric Acid (AKG)**
- **Oxaloacetate (OAA)** – Krebs cycle intermediate
- Citrulline
- D-ribose
- Creatine is a nonessential amino acid that can be synthesized from glycine, arginine, and methionine amino acids.
- calcium pyruvate
- microencapsulated NADH (NADH is the reduced form of NAD+) can be synthesized from vitamin B3 (nicotinic acid, tryptophan, nicotinamide mononucleotide (NMN))
- **Dichloroacetate** (challenging to find and expensive) - The primary site of action is the pyruvate dehydrogenase (PDH). It decreases lactic acid.

- **Fish oil** contains omega-3 fatty acids, particularly Eicosapentaenoic Acid (EPA) and Docosahexaenoic Acid (DHA).
  - **Activation of PGC-1α**: Like MCFAs, omega-3 fatty acids can also activate PGC-1α, promoting mitochondrial biogenesis and improving cellular energy capacity.
  - **Membrane Fluidity**: DHA and EPA are incorporated into mitochondrial membranes, improving their fluidity and function. It can enhance the efficiency of the electron transport chain and ATP production.
  - **Protection Against Oxidative Damage**: Omega-3 fatty acids can protect mitochondrial membranes from oxidative damage, preserving their integrity and function.

Lifestyle Modifications

Incorporating lifestyle changes can further support mitochondrial health.

- **Exercise** - Regular physical activity, particularly aerobic exercise, promotes mitochondrial biogenesis and enhances mitochondrial function. Customizing an exercise regimen to individual capabilities can help Long COVID patients improve their energy levels and overall well-being. Could you do what you can? Please don't overdo it. Use a pacing strategy, slow and steady increase in amounts.
- **Sleep Hygiene** - Quality sleep is vital for mitochondrial health and overall recovery. Establishing a regular sleep schedule and creating a conducive sleep environment can help mitigate the impact of mitochondrial dysfunction.

Stress Management

Chronic stress can adversely influence mitochondrial function. Incorporating stress management techniques—*e.g.,* mindfulness, meditation, and yoga—can minimize stress and support mitochondrial health.

Dr. Groysman's Mitochondrial 4-Step Protocol

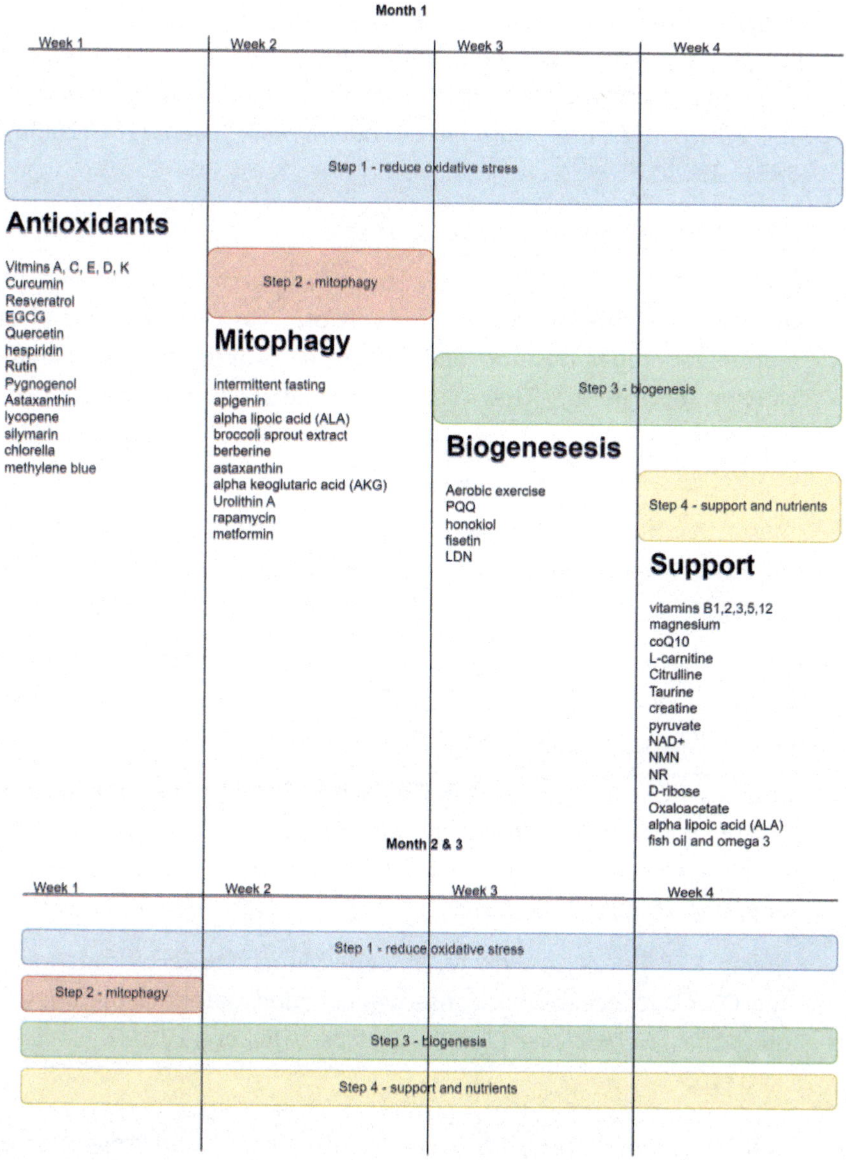
Month 1
Week 1
Week 2
Week 3
Week 4
Step 1 - reduce oxidative stress
Antioxidants
Vitmins A, C, E, D, K
Curcumin
Resveratrol
EGCG
Quercetin
hespiridin
Rutin
Pygnogenol
Astaxanthin
lycopene
silymarin
chlorella
methylene blue
Step 2 - mitophagy
Mitophagy
intermittent fasting
apigenin
alpha lipoic acid (ALA)
broccoli sprout extract
berberine
astaxanthin
alpha keoglutaric acid (AKG)
Urolithin A
rapamycin
metformin
Step 3 - biogenesis
Biogenesesis
Aerobic exercise
PQQ
honokiol
fisetin
LDN
Step 4 - support and nutrients
Support
vitamins B1,2,3,5,12
magnesium
coQ10
L-carnitine
Citrulline
Taurine
creatine
pyruvate
NAD+
NMN
NR
D-ribose
Oxaloacetate
alpha lipoic acid (ALA)
fish oil and omega 3
Month 2 & 3
Week 1
Week 2
Week 3
Week 4
Step 1 - reduce oxidative stress
Step 2 - mitophagy
Step 3 - biogenesis
Step 4 - support and nutrients

References:

1. Wang, P., Ma, J., Kim, Y. C., +10, & Hwang, P. M. (2023). WASF3 disrupts mitochondrial respiration and may mediate exercise intolerance in myalgic encephalomyelitis/chronic fatigue syndrome. *Proceedings of the National Academy of Sciences*, 120(34), e2302738120.

   https://DOI.org/10.1073/pnas.2302738120

2. Stepien KM, Cufflin N, Donald A, Jones S, Church H, Hargreaves IP. Secondary Mitochondrial Dysfunction as a Cause of Neurodegenerative Dysfunction in Lysosomal Storage Diseases and an Overview of Potential Therapies. *International Journal of Molecular Sciences*. 2022; 23(18):10573. https://DOI.org/10.3390/ijms231810573

3. Zong, Y., Li, H., Liao, P. *et al.* Mitochondrial dysfunction: mechanisms and advances in therapy. *Sig Transduct Target Ther* **9**, 124 (2024). https://DOI.org/10.1038/s41392-024-01839-8

4. Hong S, Kim S, Kim K, Lee H. Clinical Approaches for Mitochondrial Diseases. *Cells*. 2023; 12(20):2494. https://DOI.org/10.3390/cells12202494

5. Edmonds JL, Kirse DJ, Kearns D, Deutsch R, Spruijt L, Naviaux RK. The Otolaryngological Manifestations of Mitochondrial Disease and the Risk of Neurodegeneration With Infection. *Arch Otolaryngol Head Neck Surg.* 2002;128(4):355–362. DOI:10.1001/archotol.128.4.355

6. Molnar, T., Lehoczki, A., Fekete, M. *et al.* Mitochondrial dysfunction in Long COVID: mechanisms, consequences, and potential therapeutic approaches. *GeroScience* (2024). https://DOI.org/10.1007/s11357-024-01165-5

7. Chen TH, Chang CJ, Hung PH. Possible Pathogenesis and Prevention of Long COVID: SARS-CoV-2-Induced Mitochondrial Disorder. Int J Mol Sci. 2023 Apr 28;24(9):8034. DOI: 10.3390/ijms24098034. PMID: 37175745; PMCID: PMC10179190.

8. Appelman, B., Charlton, B.T., Goulding, R.P. *et al.* Muscle abnormalities worsen after post-exertional malaise in Long COVID. *Nat Commun* **15**, 17 (2024).

https://DOI.org/10.1038/s41467-023-44432-3

9. https://www.statnews.com/2023/08/09/Long-COVID-mitochondria-sars-cov-2/

10. https://theconversation.com/Long-COVID-damaged-mitochondria-in-muscles-might-be-linked-to-some-of-the-symptoms-220821

11. https://www.nih.gov/news-events/nih-research-matters/sars-cov-2-can-cause-lasting-damage-cells-energy-production

12. Wang, P., Ma, J., Kim, Y.-C., +10, & Hwang, P. M. (2023). WASF3 disrupts mitochondrial respiration and may mediate exercise intolerance in myalgic encephalomyelitis/chronic fatigue syndrome. *Proceedings of the National Academy of Sciences*, 120(34), e2302738120.

https://DOI.org/10.1073/pnas.2302738120

13. Stacpoole, P. W., Kurtz, T. L., Han, Z., & Langaee, T. (2008). Role of dichloroacetate in the treatment of genetic mitochondrial diseases. *Advanced Drug Delivery Reviews*, 60(13-14), 1476-1483. https://DOI.org/10.1016/j.addr.2008.02.014

14. Gowayed MA, Mahmoud SA, El-Sayed Y, Abu-Samra N, Kamel MA. Enhanced mitochondrial biogenesis is associated with the ameliorative action of creatine supplementation in rat soleus and cardiac muscles. Exp Ther Med. 2020 Jan;19(1):384-392. DOI: 10.3892/etm.2019.8173. Epub 2019 Nov 7. PMID: 31853315; PMCID: PMC6909667.

15. Lewis Luján LM, McCarty MF, Di Nicolantonio JJ, Gálvez Ruiz JC, Rosas-Burgos EC, Plascencia-Jatomea M, Iloki Assanga SB. Nutraceuticals/Drugs Promoting Mitophagy and Mitochondrial Biogenesis May Combat the Mitochondrial Dysfunction Driving Progression of Dry Age-Related Macular Degeneration. Nutrients. 2022 May 9;14(9):1985. DOI: 10.3390/nu14091985. PMID: 35565950; PMCID: PMC9104458.

Dysautonomia in Long COVID

Dysautonomia is a disorder of the *autonomic nervous system (ANS), and it can manifest in a range of symptoms that affect* heart rate, BP, digestion, and temperature regulation. This chapter delves into the mechanisms of dysautonomia in Long COVID and explores potential treatment strategies.

The Autonomic Nervous System

The ANS regulates involuntary physiological processes such as heart rate, BP, respiration, digestion, and temperature control. It comprises two main branches:

- **Sympathetic Nervous System (SNS)**: Prepares the body for "*fight or flight*" responses.

- **Parasympathetic Nervous System (PNS)**: Promotes "rest and digest" activities.

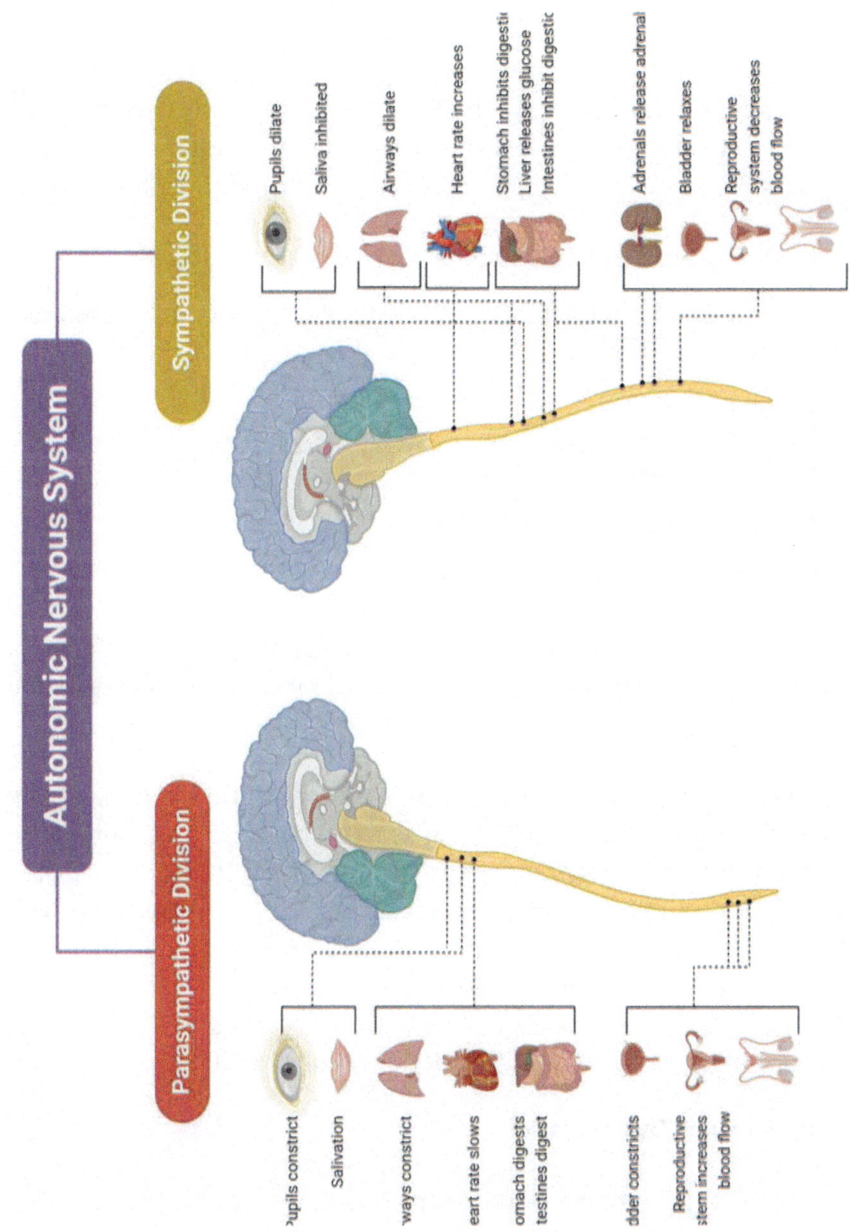
Autonomic Nervous System
Sympathetic Division
Pupils dilate
Saliva inhibited
Airways dilate
Heart rate increases
Stomach inhibits digesti
Liver releases glucose
Intestines inhibit digestic
Adrenals release adrenal
Bladder relaxes
Reproductive system decreases blood flow
Parasympathetic Division
upils constrict
Salivation
ways constrict
eart rate slows
omach digests
testines digest
dder constricts
Reproductive
stem increases
blood flow

What is Dysautonomia?

Dysautonomia refers to a dysfunction of the ANS, which leads to an imbalance between the SNS and PNS. It can result from various conditions, including viral infections. Symptoms can vary extensively but often include:

- Tachycardia or bradycardia
- Orthostatic intolerance or Postural Orthostatic Tachycardia Syndrome (POTS)
- BP fluctuations
- Gastrointestinal disturbances
- Temperature regulation issues
- Fatigue and exercise intolerance

Dysautonomia can develop an overactive sympathetic nervous system, leading to a persistent *fight or flight* situation, or it can affect a vagus nerve dysfunction.

Emerging evidence indicates that SARS-CoV-2 can impact the ANS, leading to dysautonomia. It may be due to direct viral effects on autonomic pathways, vagus nerve thickening and damage, immune-mediated damage, or persistent inflammatory responses. Long COVID patients with dysautonomia may experience a broad array of debilitating symptoms, complicating their recovery process.

Mechanisms that can cause Dysautonomia in Long COVID

1. **Immune Dysregulation**

    - The immune response to SARS-CoV-2 can result in cytokine release and inflammation, potentially damaging autonomic pathways and leading to dysautonomia. Continued immune activation and autoantibody production may further exacerbate autonomic dysfunction.

2. **Direct Viral Impact**

   - SARS-CoV-2 may directly infect and damage neurons or glial cells involved in autonomic regulation. Viral particles have been detected in the brain and other tissues, suggesting a direct impact on the ANS.

3. **Vascular and Endothelial Dysfunction**

   - COVID-19-associated endothelial damage and microvascular dysfunction can impair blood flow and autonomic regulation. It can contribute to symptoms such as orthostatic intolerance and POTS.

4. **Serotonin deficiency**

   a. **Serotonin Gut Production:** About 90-95% of the body's serotonin is produced in the gut, regulating bowel movements and motility. It is produced by immune cells in the gut, nerve endings, and specialized cells in the gut called enterochromaffin cells. It is associated with the gut-brain axis and relies on the microbiome interactions for successful production. Serotonin deficiency in the gut can lead to gastrointestinal issues, which are common in dysautonomia.

   b. **Vagus Nerve Dysfunction:** The vagus nerve—a significant component of the ANS—communicates between the gut and the brain. Serotonin plays a vital role in this communication, and deficiencies can disrupt this pathway, affecting autonomic regulation.

Postural Orthostatic Tachycardia Syndrome (POTS)

POTS is a form of dysautonomia; its hallmark is orthostasis, which is intolerance to standing or being upright. The intolerance comes in the form of dizziness or tachycardia. It is typically due to prolonged sinus tachycardia, which increases heart rate. An increase in heart rate is typical and expected in response to standing due to a temporary drop in blood volume available to the heart due to gravity. The arteries in the lower extremities will contract and squeeze the blood back up towards the heart. It happens quickly after standing when your ANS is functioning normally. However, this mechanism is sluggish in POTS and takes over 10 minutes.

Orthostatic Hypotension (OH) is a more severe form of POTS. The arteries in the lower extremities cannot squeeze down at all, leading to a significant drop in blood pressure when standing. It can lead to dizziness and fainting because insufficient blood flow gets to the brain.

POTS is relatively easy to diagnose using a lean or tilt table test. What happens if you have orthostatic intolerance but do not meet the criteria of POTS as outlined below? You still treat the orthostasis the same way.

To summarize, for POTS to be diagnosed, you need the heart rate to increase at or after 10 minutes by 30 beats or more while upright or standing. However, blood pressure is not used to diagnose POTS.

If the blood pressure falls while standing in the first few minutes, it may be orthostatic hypotension (OH), which overrides the POTS diagnosis. OH is just a more severe case of POTS. It is either POTS or OH, not both, and they are mutually exclusive.

Hemodynamic criteria for conditions causing orthostatic intolerance

Diagnosis	**Fall in systolic – top number for BP (SBP) upon standing**	**Fall in DBP (bottom number) upon standing**	**Increase in HR upon standing**	**Timing**
Orthostatic Hypotension	≥ 20 mmHg	≥ 10 mmHg	Not specified	Sustained BP fall within 3 min standing
POTS	SBP fall not meeting OH criteria	DBP fall not meeting OH criteria	> by 30 bpm or > 120 bpm	Sustained HR increase within 10 min standing

Abbreviations: OH = orthostatic hypotension, SBP = systolic blood pressure (top number), DBP = diastolic blood pressure (bottom number), BP = blood pressure, HR = heart rate, POTS = postural orthostatic tachycardia syndrome

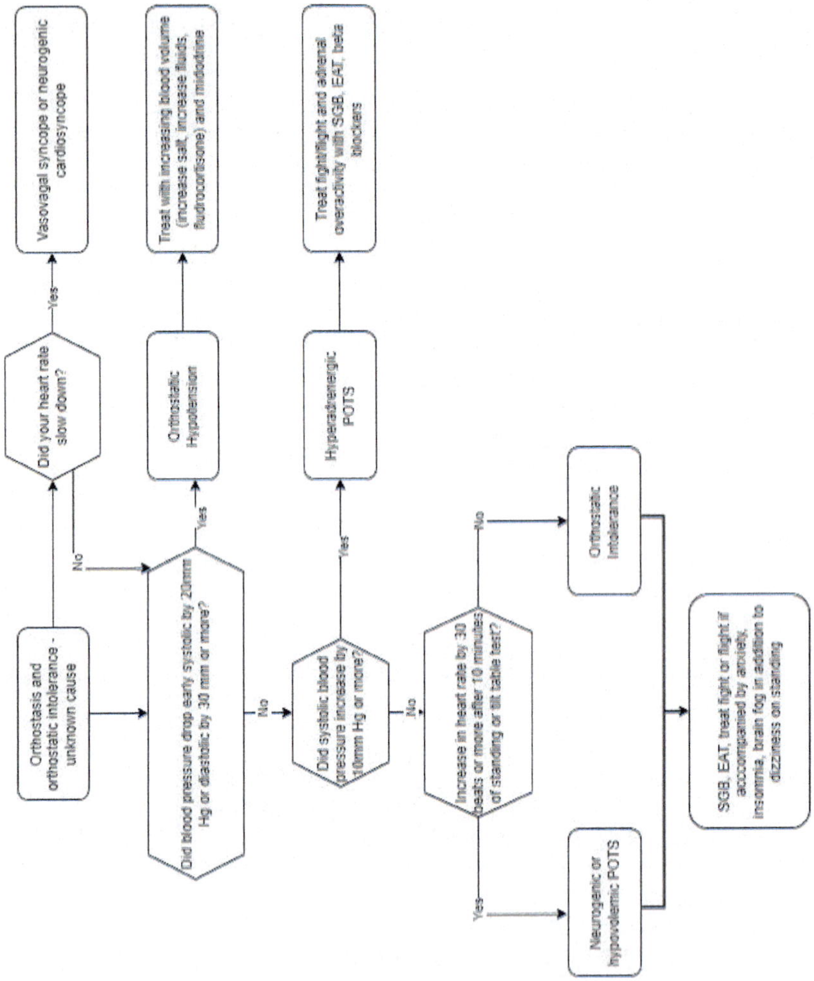

What exactly is orthostatic intolerance?

Let's take a closer look at orthostatic intolerance. What is it? It is dizziness to the point of passing out, and this condition is created when the brain doesn't get enough blood flow when standing or remaining upright. Orthostatic intolerance can occur for several reasons. In POTS, the heart rate is the problem. Because the blood vessels in your legs and abdomen cannot adjust fast enough after you stand, blood tends to pool in gravity-dependent areas, such as your legs. Consequently, the heart experiences less blood volume coming in, so it speeds up and pumps harder to increase the blood flow. Therefore, it causes palpitations, chest pain, and dizziness.

The blood flow is eventually restored; the arteries and veins become sluggish.

A more severe form of POTS is orthostatic hypotension, where not only the heart rate increases, but the BP drops. The blood vessels in the legs cannot respond at all to constrict and force the blood to the heart. It causes the BP to drop. Both the BP and the heart rate are responsible for the symptoms.

Sometimes, it is a combination of the increased heart rate and the low BP that cause the symptoms but do not meet the criteria to diagnose either POTS or orthostatic hypotension. In those cases, we just call it orthostatic intolerance. It is still accurate and causes symptoms.

> *We had a patient come in with a diagnosis of POTS but no orthostatic intolerance. Despite a diagnostic increase in heart rate of 30 beats or more, which led to the diagnosis of POTS, there was no orthostasis. This patient was already on beta blockers. What would the next step be?*

Strategies for Treating POTS in Long COVID

Treatments are geared towards treating the symptoms by decreasing heart rate to reduce tachycardia and increasing blood pressure. I generally prefer to treat the dysautonomia as a whole rather than just POTS, but I may utilize these treatments temporarily to help with symptoms until I can address the dysautonomia itself.

- Stellate ganglion block
- Epipharyngeal Abrasive Treatment (EAT)

Symptomatic treatment

Heart rate reducers

- **Beta-Blockers:** Beta-blockers, such as propranolol, can help manage tachycardia and reduce sympathetic overactivity. They can be particularly beneficial for patients with POTS. Beta-blockers can also lower your BP by dilating your arteries. Remarkably, beta-blockers can hamper exercising and increase fatigue due to the same heart rate-lowering effect.

- **Ivabradine (Corlinor):** targets the sinoatrial node to reduce heart rate without affecting BP, making it helpful in managing Inappropriate Sinus Tachycardia (IST) in Long COVID patients.

Blood Pressure Increasers

- **Fludrocortisone:** Fludrocortisone, a mineralocorticoid, can increase blood volume and improve orthostatic tolerance by promoting sodium and water retention. It is often used in patients with orthostatic hypotension.

- **Midodrine:** Midodrine is an alpha-adrenergic agonist that increases vascular tone and BP, helping to alleviate symptoms of orthostatic hypotension and POTS.

- **Increasing blood volume:** Increasing fluid and salt intake can help expand blood volume and enhance orthostatic tolerance. Moreover, patients are often advised to drink at least 2-3 liters of water daily and consume additional salt.
    - **Hydration**
    - **Salt Intake (salt is salt and is also an electrolyte).**
    - **Compression Garments** - Wearing compression stockings with abdominal binders can improve venous return and reduce orthostatic symptoms. These garments help prevent blood pooling in the lower extremities.
    - **Postural Maneuvers**
        - crossing legs while standing
        - tensing leg muscles
        - lying down when feeling

Other treatments for POTS

- **Physical Exercise** - Graded exercise programs can improve cardiovascular conditioning and autonomic function, starting with low-intensity activities and gradually increasing. Exercises like recumbent cycling, swimming, and walking are recommended. Use pacing to try to avoid crashes and post-exertional malaise.

- **Dietary Modifications** - Eating small, frequent meals and avoiding large carbohydrate-rich meals can help stabilize BP and reduce gastrointestinal symptoms. Some patients benefit from a low-histamine or anti-inflammatory diet.

- **Sleep Hygiene** - Ensuring adequate and quality sleep is crucial for autonomic regulation. Most of the repairs occur during deep sleep. Therefore, establishing a regular sleep schedule, creating a restful sleep ecosystem, and addressing sleep disorders is essential.

- **Stress Management** - Chronic stress can exacerbate autonomic dysfunction. Techniques such as mindfulness, meditation, yoga, and deep-breathing exercises can help manage stress and improve ANS balance.

- **Biofeedback** - Biofeedback techniques can help patients better control their autonomic responses by providing real-time feedback on physiological functions like heart rate and breathing.

References:

1. Fedorowski, A., Sutton, R. Autonomic dysfunction and postural orthostatic tachycardia syndrome in post-acute COVID-19 syndrome. *Nat Rev Cardiol* **20**, 281–282 (2023). https://doi.org/10.1038/s41569-023-00842-w

2. Ormiston CK, Świątkiewicz I, Taub PR. Postural orthostatic tachycardia syndrome as a sequela of COVID-19. Heart Rhythm.

2022 Nov;19(11):1880-1889. doi: 10.1016/j.hrthm.2022.07.014. Epub 2022 Jul 16. PMID: 35853576; PMCID: PMC9287587.

3. Mallick D, Goyal L, Chourasia P, Zapata MR, Yashi K, Surani S. COVID-19 Induced Postural Orthostatic Tachycardia Syndrome (POTS): A Review. Cureus. 2023 Mar 31;15(3):e36955. doi: 10.7759/cureus.36955. PMID: 37009342; PMCID: PMC10065129.

4. Chadda, K. R., Blakey, E. E., Huang, C. L.-H., & Jeevaratnam, K. (2022). Long COVID-19 and postural orthostatic tachycardia syndrome—Is dysautonomia to be blamed? *Frontiers in Cardiovascular Medicine*, 9, 860198. https://doi.org/10.3389/fcvm.2022.860198

Accelerated Aging

You may have noticed that you may look older than usual or that you have aged faster than you have before Long COVID. There is a reason for this. There are two factors in play:

1. Dysautonomia and chronic fight/flight state

2. Mitochondria dysfunction, this includes oxidative stress, telomere shortening, methylation, histone modifications, and epigenics.

Aging appears to be caused by a number of normal and abnormal processes. It has to do with being able to heal and repair tissues which is a state created by a prominent parasympathetic nervous system. **Deep sleep** is where this system shines, but repair and healing should happen throughout the day.

Aging Faster than chronological age in long covid occurs for **3 reasons:**

1) People who have **dysautonomia** are stuck in fight/flight. Your body has to prioritize between healing and digesting and fighting for your survival. When you are **stuck in fight/flight**, your body's focus is mostly on survival. During deep sleep, stage 3 sleep, your body is supposed to be focused nearly 100% on healing. During healing, your stem cells can divide, repair tissue, and replace tissues. This is a very important part of healing overnight. <u>If you don't fix fight-/flight first, the rest won't matter since healing and repair is significantly slowed or stopped.</u>

2) People with **mitochondrial dysfunction** are also under a constant **oxidative stress**. Normally, our bodies can just balance the oxidative stress with internal antioxidants. Under any chronic illness, the oxidative stress is greater. Controlling the oxidative stress is critical to stopping the accelerated aging.

3) Many of the other processes like **epigenics**, **gene methylation**, **telomere** length, and **senescence** are all linked to mitochondrial mechanisms.

What Causes Accelerated Aging and What You Can Do about it?

If you just try to cram in a bunch of stem cell treatments into you, you won't get a good result if you are not already in healing mode. Want to know more? Read on!

Mechanisms of Aging

1. **Telomere Shortening**

   - **What it is:** Telomeres are protective caps at the ends of chromosomes. Every time a cell divides, telomeres shorten. Once they become too short, the cell enters a state called **senescence** or dies. This happens because the cell has lost its ability to divide and function.

   - **Impact:** As more cells enter senescence or die, tissue repair and regeneration slow down, contributing to the signs of aging.

2. **Mitochondrial Dysfunction**

   - **What it is:** Mitochondria are the "powerhouses" of the cell, generating energy (ATP) necessary for cellular functions. Over time, mitochondrial DNA (mtDNA) becomes damaged, leading to less efficient energy production and an increase in **reactive oxygen species (ROS)**, or free radicals, that damage cells.

- **Impact:** This leads to energy deficits in cells and contributes to aging-related diseases like neurodegeneration and muscle weakness.

3. **Accumulation of Senescent Cells**

- **What it is:** Senescent cells are damaged cells that stop dividing but don't die. They release inflammatory signals known as the **senescence-associated secretory phenotype (SASP)**, which damages nearby healthy cells.

- **Impact:** The accumulation of these cells in tissues is associated with chronic inflammation and aging-related diseases such as cancer and cardiovascular conditions.

4. **Loss of Proteostasis:** refers to the body's ability to maintain proper protein folding and degradation. With age, this balance is disrupted, leading to the accumulation of misfolded or damaged proteins, which can lead to diseases like **Alzheimer's** and **Parkinson's**. Abnormal proteins don't fold correctly. Amino acid mutations and substitutions can also cause this. This is covered more in the *Complete Long COVID Handbook: Mitochondria, Volume 3.*

5. **Epigenetic Alterations**

- **Epigenetics** involves changes in gene expression without altering the underlying DNA sequence. Age-related changes in epigenetic markers, like **DNA methylation** and **histone modification**, disrupt normal gene function, leading to the dysregulation of cellular processes.

- **Impact:** This contributes to the loss of cellular identity and functionality, promoting aging and disease.

6. **Stem Cell Exhaustion**

    - **What it is:** Stem cells are responsible for regenerating tissues. Over time, their capacity to regenerate declines due to damage or exhaustion, leading to impaired tissue repair.

    - **Impact:** Reduced stem cell activity contributes to the weakening of tissue function and increased susceptibility to injury or illness.

7. **Deregulated Nutrient Sensing**

    - **What it is:** As we age, pathways involved in nutrient sensing, such as **insulin/IGF-1 signaling**, become less regulated. These pathways are crucial for growth, metabolism, and longevity. These are again mitochondrial.

    - **Impact:** Disrupted nutrient sensing can lead to metabolic disorders like type 2 diabetes, which are closely linked with aging.

What about Telomere Shortening?

Telomere shortening is primarily caused by the natural process of cell division and is influenced by various environmental, biological, and lifestyle factors. Telomere shortening is like a "countdown timer" inside your cells that **gets shorter every time your cells divide**.

1. What Are Telomeres?

- Imagine your DNA (the instructions for how your body works) is like a shoelace. At the ends of your shoelaces, there are little plastic tips that stop them from fraying and falling apart. Those plastic tips are like **telomeres**, and they protect your DNA every time a cell divides.

- You are born with a certain length of telomeres protecting each of your cell's chromosomes. The length depends on your genetics and environmental factors. You can't alter your telomere starting lengths at birth, but you can keep their lengths longer than usual.

2. Cell Division and Shortening

- Your body is made up of billions of tiny cells. These cells need to divide to grow, repair damage, and keep you healthy. But, every time a cell divides, the telomeres get a little bit shorter, just like cutting a tiny piece off the plastic tip of your shoelace.

- As the telomeres get shorter and shorter, they can't protect the DNA as well. Eventually, when they get too short, the cell can't divide anymore, and it either stops working or dies. This is a normal part of aging.

3. What Makes Telomeres Shorten Faster?

- Certain things can make telomeres shorten faster, like **stress**, **not enough sleep**, **bad eating habits**, or **not getting enough exercise**. <u>This is a bad thing</u>. These things put extra pressure on your cells, causing more wear and tear on the telomeres.

    - **Oxidative Stress:** Oxidative stress, which is the result of an imbalance between the production of free radicals and the body's ability to detoxify them, can accelerate telomere shortening. Free radicals can cause damage to the DNA, including the telomeres, leading to more rapid shortening.

    - **Bad life choices: Smoking, poor diet**, **obesity**, and **lack of exercise** have all been associated with increased oxidative stress and inflammation, which can lead to accelerated telomere shortening.

    - **Psychological stress**, especially chronic stress, has also been linked to shorter telomeres through stress-induced biological pathways (e.g., elevated cortisol levels, immune system dysregulation).

- **Inflammation (Chronic Inflammation):** Chronic inflammation generates pro-inflammatory molecules (cytokines) that can increase oxidative stress and tissue damage, contributing to faster telomere erosion.

- **Environmental Factors:** Exposure to **pollutants**, such as air pollution or chemicals, and **UV radiation** from excessive sun exposure, can increase oxidative stress, leading to telomere shortening.

- **Genetic Factors:** Some individuals may have genetic variations that influence the length of their telomeres and the rate at which they shorten. The enzyme **telomerase**, which can add DNA back to the ends of telomeres, plays a crucial role here. Mutations affecting telomerase function can result in faster telomere attrition.

- **Disease States:** Certain diseases, particularly those involving chronic inflammation or oxidative stress (e.g., **cardiovascular diseases**, **diabetes**, **cancer**, and **chronic infections**), are associated with accelerated telomere shortening.

- **Chronic viral infections**, such as HIV or possibly long COVID, may also increase the rate of telomere shortening due to ongoing immune system activation.

4. Why Does it Matter?

- When telomeres get really short, cells get old and can't work properly anymore. This is why telomere shortening is connected to **aging**—over time, our cells can't divide and repair as easily, which makes us look and feel older.

In short: Telomeres are like the protective caps on the ends of your DNA, and every time a cell divides, they get a bit shorter. When they get too short, the cells can't divide anymore, and that's one reason why we age.

Epigenetics

It is a really cool way to understand how your genes (which are like instructions for how your body works) can be turned **on** or **off** depending on things that happen around you. Let me break it down:

1. What Are Genes?

- Think of genes like a **recipe book** inside every cell in your body. This recipe book has all the instructions for how your body grows, looks, and works. These instructions tell your body things like what color your eyes are or how tall you might be.

2. What is Epigenetics?

- Now, imagine you have a sticky note that you can put on a page of your recipe book that says "**Don't use this recipe right now**." That's kind of what **epigenetics** does. It's not changing the recipes (the genes) themselves, but it's putting a mark on them that says whether to use them or not.

- Epigenetics is like the "switches" that tell your body which genes should be **turned on** (used) and which ones should be **turned off** (not used). This helps your body respond to things happening around you, like what you eat, how much exercise you get, or even how stressed you are.

3. How Does Epigenetics Work?

- There are special molecules, like **methyl groups**, that can stick to your DNA and tell your body to **silence** or **activate** certain genes. It's like putting those sticky notes on different parts of your recipe book.

- When these marks are added to certain genes, it can either stop the gene from doing its job or make it more active. The gene itself isn't changed, but how it's used is.

4. Why Is Epigenetics Important?

- Epigenetics explains why **identical twins** (who have the same genes) can look or act differently as they get older. Even though their DNA is the same, their epigenetic "marks" might be different because of their different life experiences.

- It's also why **your environment**—like how much sleep you get, whether you smoke, or how healthy your diet is—can affect your body. These things can change your epigenetic "marks" and impact how your genes work, which can affect your health, energy levels, or even how you age.

5. Can Epigenetics Be Inherited?

- Interestingly, some epigenetic changes can be passed down from parents to children. For example, if your parents had a tough time with food or were exposed to certain things in their environment, that could leave marks on their genes, and some of those marks might be passed down to you.

6. Why It's Like a Dimmer Switch

- If genes are like light bulbs, epigenetics is the **dimmer switch** that controls how bright the light shines. Instead of just turning genes on or off like a regular switch, epigenetics can control how **strong** or **weak** a gene's activity is—like making the light brighter or dimmer.

Fight/Flight and Aging

As people age, the balance between the sympathetic and parasympathetic systems can shift, often favoring sympathetic dominance, especially in those with chronic stress or dysautonomia. This has several implications for aging.

Chronic sympathetic activation drives everything else. This leads to **oxidative stress, inflammation**, and **DNA damage**, all of which accelerate biological aging. It also impairs the body's ability to repair and regenerate tissues, contributing to degenerative conditions like cardiovascular disease and cognitive decline.

In Long COVID, healing and repair can't happen because most everyone is stuck in fight/flight mode. This locks you in in chronic stress too. You can't heal or repair while in this mode. Reversing this state is important before you can reverse the accelerated aging and the mitochondrial problems.

1. **Chronic Sympathetic Activation (Fight or Flight)**
    - When the sympathetic nervous system is persistently activated, as seen in dysautonomia, the body remains in a heightened state of stress, with elevated levels of Epinephrine (**adrenaline)** and **cortisol**. Chronic stress can:
        - **Suppress the immune system**: Prolonged cortisol release reduces immune function, making it harder for the body to respond to infections or tissue damage.
        - **Inhibit tissue repair**: The body prioritizes short-term survival over long-term maintenance during fight or flight. As a result, processes like wound healing and cellular repair are delayed.
        - **Increase inflammation**: While acute inflammation is part of healing, chronic sympathetic activation can lead to persistent low-grade inflammation, contributing to tissue damage and impairing the healing response.

2. **Impact on Rest and Digest (Parasympathetic Activity)**

    - The parasympathetic nervous system is crucial for healing, digestion, and recovery. It promotes functions like cellular repair, nutrient absorption, and immune regulation. In dysautonomia, if the parasympathetic system is underactive, these essential healing processes are compromised.

    - **Vagus nerve dysfunction**, a key component of parasympathetic activity, is common in dysautonomia and can prevent the body from entering a restful state conducive to healing.

Mitochondria and Aging

Mitochondria play a central role in longevity and anti-aging processes due to their essential function in cellular energy production, metabolic regulation, and oxidative stress management. These organelles generate ATP (adenosine triphosphate) through oxidative phosphorylation, which powers nearly all cellular activities. However, mitochondrial function tends to decline with age, leading to reduced energy production, increased oxidative stress, and subsequent cellular damage. This dysfunction is a hallmark of aging and is linked to many age-related diseases, including neurodegenerative disorders, cardiovascular disease, and metabolic conditions.

Key concepts connecting mitochondria with longevity and anti-aging.

1. Mitochondrial Dysfunction and Aging

- Mitochondria generate reactive oxygen species (ROS) as byproducts of energy production. Over time, an excess of ROS can lead to oxidative damage to mitochondrial DNA (mtDNA), proteins, and lipids, which impairs mitochondrial function. This process contributes to cellular aging and age-related diseases.

- Mitochondrial DNA mutations accumulate with age, further impairing mitochondrial function, which in turn can trigger cellular senescence (a state where cells lose their ability to divide and function properly).

2. Mitophagy and Mitochondrial Quality Control

- Mitophagy is the process of selectively degrading damaged mitochondria. Efficient mitophagy is crucial for maintaining mitochondrial health. As we age, mitophagy declines, leading to the accumulation of dysfunctional mitochondria, which contributes to aging and degenerative diseases.

- Enhancing mitophagy is seen as a potential therapeutic strategy to combat aging. Interventions like calorie restriction (intermittent fasting) and certain compounds (e.g., spermidine) are believed to promote mitophagy and improve mitochondrial function.

3. NAD+ and Mitochondrial Function

- NAD+ (nicotinamide adenine dinucleotide) is a vital coenzyme in mitochondrial energy production and repair processes. NAD+ levels decline with age, which affects mitochondrial efficiency and cellular metabolism.

- NAD+ boosters, such as **nicotinamide riboside (NR)** and **nicotinamide mononucleotide (NMN)**, are being studied for their potential to restore mitochondrial function, improve cellular metabolism, and extend lifespan. These precursors help enhance mitochondrial biogenesis (the formation of new mitochondria) and repair, improving overall energy production and reducing age-related metabolic decline.

4. Sirtuins and Mitochondrial Health

- **Sirtuins** are a family of proteins that regulate mitochondrial function, stress responses, and metabolism. The most well-known,

SIRT1, is activated by NAD+ and influences pathways involved in longevity, such as those triggered by calorie restriction or exercise.

- SIRT1 activates **PGC-1α** (peroxisome proliferator-activated receptor gamma coactivator 1-alpha), which promotes mitochondrial biogenesis and enhances the cell's ability to handle oxidative stress. Boosting sirtuin activity is seen as a promising anti-aging intervention.

5. Caloric Restriction and Mitochondrial Efficiency

- Caloric restriction (CR), which involves reducing calorie intake without malnutrition, is one of the most well-researched methods for extending lifespan. CR improves mitochondrial function by enhancing mitochondrial biogenesis, reducing oxidative stress, and improving energy efficiency. It triggers pathways involving **AMPK, mTOR**, and sirtuins, all of which are linked to longevity and mitochondrial health.

6. Mitochondrial Biogenesis and Exercise

- Physical activity, particularly endurance exercise, stimulates mitochondrial biogenesis by activating pathways like **AMP-activated protein kinase (AMPK)** and PGC-1α. This enhances mitochondrial capacity and efficiency, helping maintain energy production and metabolic health with age.

- Exercise also reduces mitochondrial ROS production, supporting longevity by lowering oxidative damage.

7. Mitochondrial Targeted Antioxidants

- Antioxidants like **coenzyme Q10 (CoQ10)**, **mitoquidone (MitoQ)**, and **skQ1** are designed to specifically target mitochondria and reduce oxidative stress. These compounds are being explored for their potential to protect against mitochondrial damage and extend health span.

8. Fisetin and Senolytics

- **Senolytics** are compounds that target and eliminate senescent cells, which accumulate with age and contribute to tissue dysfunction. Fisetin, a flavonoid found in fruits like strawberries, has been studied for its senolytic properties. By removing senescent cells, senolytics may improve mitochondrial function and extend health span.

Oxidative stress

It plays a central role in the aging process and is a key contributor to the development of age-related diseases. Here's how oxidative stress is related to aging:

1. What is Oxidative Stress?

- Oxidative stress occurs when there's an imbalance between **free radicals** (reactive oxygen species, ROS) and the body's ability to neutralize them with **antioxidants**. Free radicals are highly reactive molecules with unpaired electrons that can damage cells, proteins, lipids, and DNA.

- While free radicals are naturally produced as byproducts of normal cellular metabolism (especially in the mitochondria), excessive levels can overwhelm the body's antioxidant defenses.

2. Role in Aging: The Free Radical Theory

- The **free radical theory of aging**, proposed by Denham Harman in the 1950s, suggests that cumulative damage from oxidative stress is a major driver of aging. According to this theory, the continuous production of ROS during metabolism leads to cellular damage over time, which accelerates the aging process.

- ROS cause damage to key cellular components:

- **DNA**: Oxidative stress can lead to mutations, DNA breaks, and damage to telomeres (the protective ends of chromosomes). This contributes to cellular aging and senescence.

- **Proteins**: ROS can oxidize proteins, impairing their function and structure. Damaged proteins accumulate, leading to loss of cellular function and tissue integrity.

- **Lipids**: ROS attack lipids in cell membranes, a process called **lipid peroxidation**, which disrupts membrane integrity and impairs cell signaling.

3. Mitochondrial Dysfunction and Aging

- Mitochondria, the energy-producing organelles of the cell, are a major source of ROS, as oxidative phosphorylation (energy production) generates free radicals as a byproduct.

- Over time, mitochondrial DNA (mtDNA) becomes damaged by ROS, leading to dysfunction in the mitochondria. This creates a vicious cycle, as dysfunctional mitochondria produce even more ROS, further exacerbating cellular damage.

- Mitochondrial dysfunction is closely linked to many aging-related processes, including the decline in energy metabolism and increased susceptibility to diseases like neurodegeneration, cardiovascular diseases, and metabolic disorders.

4. Oxidative Stress and Cellular Senescence

- Chronic oxidative damage can push cells into a state of **cellular senescence**, where they permanently stop dividing. Senescent cells accumulate with age and secrete pro-inflammatory molecules (the **senescence-associated secretory phenotype**, or SASP), which contributes to tissue dysfunction and chronic inflammation, often referred to as **inflammaging**.

5. Telomere Shortening

- Oxidative stress accelerates telomere shortening, which is a key marker of aging. Shortened telomeres signal the cell to enter senescence or undergo apoptosis (cell death), reducing the regenerative capacity of tissues over time.

6. Age-Related Diseases

Oxidative stress is implicated in many age-related diseases:

- **Cardiovascular disease**: Oxidative stress damages blood vessels and contributes to atherosclerosis, the buildup of plaques in the arteries.

- **Neurodegenerative diseases**: ROS play a role in the development of conditions like Alzheimer's and Parkinson's disease by damaging neurons and promoting neuroinflammation.

- **Cancer**: Oxidative stress can induce DNA mutations, contributing to the transformation of normal cells into cancerous cells.

- **Diabetes**: Chronic oxidative stress impairs insulin signaling and contributes to the complications of diabetes, such as kidney and nerve damage.

- **Chronic inflammation**: As oxidative damage accumulates, the immune system responds with chronic, low-grade inflammation, which further drives aging and disease progression.

7. Antioxidants and Aging

- The body naturally produces antioxidants (e.g., glutathione, superoxide dismutase, catalase) to counteract ROS. However, as we age, the body's natural antioxidant defenses decline, making cells more susceptible to oxidative damage.

- **Dietary antioxidants** (e.g., vitamin C, vitamin E, polyphenols) from fruits, vegetables, and other foods can help reduce oxidative stress by neutralizing free radicals.

- Some research suggests that maintaining a balance between free radicals and antioxidants can help slow down the aging process and reduce the risk of age-related diseases, although the effectiveness of antioxidant supplementation in humans is still debated.

8. Interventions to Mitigate Oxidative Stress and Aging

- **Healthy diet**: A diet rich in antioxidants (e.g., fruits, vegetables, nuts, and whole grains) can help reduce oxidative stress.

- **Regular exercise**: Exercise promotes the production of endogenous antioxidants and helps improve mitochondrial efficiency. However, excessive exercise can increase ROS, so balance is key.

- **Caloric restriction**: Caloric restriction (or intermittent fasting) has been shown to reduce oxidative stress and promote longevity in various animal studies, partly by reducing mitochondrial ROS production.

- **Sleep**: Adequate sleep is essential for maintaining proper antioxidant function and mitigating oxidative stress.

- **Stress management**: Chronic psychological stress can increase ROS production, so managing stress through practices like mindfulness, yoga, and relaxation techniques is beneficial.

Potential Anti-Aging Therapies

1. **Telomere Extension Therapies**

    - **Approach:** Therapies that aim to extend telomeres using **telomerase activation**. Telomerase is an enzyme that can lengthen telomeres, potentially allowing cells to divide for longer periods without entering senescence.

- **Research:** Some studies, including gene therapy and compounds like **TA-65**, suggest that telomerase activation may extend lifespan in animal models. However, long-term human efficacy is still being studied.

2. **Senolytics**

- **Approach:** These are drugs that selectively eliminate senescent cells. By clearing out these damaged cells, senolytics can reduce inflammation and promote tissue regeneration.

- **Examples: Dasatinib** and **quercetin** are examples of senolytic drugs that have shown promise in reducing age-related conditions and improving physical function in animal studies and small human trials.

3. **Mitochondrial Enhancement**

- **Approach:** Improving mitochondrial function can enhance energy production and reduce oxidative damage. Therapies include antioxidants, mitochondrial-targeted nutrients, and drugs like **NAD+ precursors** (e.g., **nicotinamide riboside** or **NMN**).

- **Research:** NAD+ boosters have been linked to improved mitochondrial function and may help delay aging by supporting cellular repair mechanisms.

4. **Caloric Restriction and Fasting**

- **Approach: Caloric restriction (CR)** and **intermittent fasting** have been shown to extend lifespan in various animal models by reducing oxidative stress, improving metabolism, and promoting autophagy (the body's process of clearing out damaged cells).

- **Research:** Studies in humans suggest that CR can lower markers of aging, such as insulin resistance and inflammation, but long-term effects on lifespan are still being investigated.

5. **Epigenetic Reprogramming**

- **Approach:** Epigenetic therapies aim to reverse age-related changes in gene expression by resetting the epigenome. For instance, **Yamanaka factors**, a set of genes that can revert cells to a more youthful state, have been studied for their potential to reprogram aging cells.

- **Research:** Early studies in mice have shown promise in rejuvenating tissues and extending lifespan, but human applications are still in experimental stages.

6. **Stem Cell Therapy**

- **Approach:** Replacing or rejuvenating old stem cells with healthy ones can improve tissue repair and regeneration. Techniques like **mesenchymal stem cell (MSC) therapy** are being explored to treat age-related diseases.

- **Research:** Some clinical trials show improvements in immune function and inflammation, but widespread use of stem cell therapy for aging is not yet fully established.

7. **Drugs Targeting Nutrient Sensing Pathways**

- **Approach:** Modulating nutrient-sensing pathways, such as **mTOR** (mechanistic target of rapamycin) and **AMPK** (AMP-activated protein kinase), can mimic the effects of caloric restriction and improve longevity.

- **Examples: Rapamycin** is an mTOR inhibitor that has been shown to extend lifespan in animal models. **Metformin**, a diabetes drug, is also being studied for its potential anti-aging effects by improving insulin sensitivity and reducing inflammation.

8. **Lifestyle and Dietary Interventions**

   - **Exercise:** Regular physical activity is associated with improved mitochondrial function, reduced inflammation, and enhanced cellular repair mechanisms.
   - **Diet:** Diets rich in antioxidants (e.g., vitamins C and E), healthy fats, and nutrient-dense foods may help counteract oxidative damage and inflammation, slowing down aging.
   - **Sleep and Stress Management:** Chronic stress and poor sleep accelerate aging by increasing inflammation and dysregulating important hormones like cortisol. Prioritizing sleep and stress reduction can promote longevity.

References:

- Srivastava, S. (2017). The mitochondrial basis of aging and age-related disorders. *Genes, 8*(12), 398. https://doi.org/10.3390/genes8120398
- Guo, Y., Guan, T., Shafiq, K., Yu, Q., Jiao, X., Na, D., Li, M., Zhang, G., & Kong, J. (2023). Mitochondrial dysfunction in aging. *Ageing Research Reviews, 88*, 101955. https://doi.org/10.1016/j.arr.2023.101955
- Rossiello, F., Jurk, D., Passos, J.F. *et al.* Telomere dysfunction in ageing and age-related diseases. *Nat Cell Biol* **24**, 135–147 (2022). https://doi.org/10.1038/s41556-022-00842-x
- Cui, H., Kong, Y., & Zhang, H. (2011). Oxidative stress, mitochondrial dysfunction, and aging. *Journal of Signal Transduction, 2012*(1), 646354. https://doi.org/10.1155/2012/646354
- Maldonado, E., Morales-Pison, S., Urbina, F., & Solari, A. (2023). Aging hallmarks and the role of oxidative stress. *Antioxidants, 12*(3), 651. https://doi.org/10.3390/antiox12030651

Chronic Fatigue Syndrome (ME/CFS)

Chronic Fatigue Syndrome—also known as *Myalgic Encephalomyelitis* (ME/CFS)—is a complex and debilitating condition characterized by extreme fatigue that cannot be improved with rest and worsens with physical or mental activity. While there is no known cure for ME/CFS, different medications can help manage symptoms and improve the quality of life for those affected. I mention it because many symptoms and mechanisms also occur in Long COVID. This chapter explores the different types of medications commonly used to treat ME/CFS symptoms, how they work, and considerations for their use. Because Long COVID shares many aspects of ME/CFS, reviewing the available treatment options is prudent. It is important to determine if you are suffering from ME/CFS or a chronic fatigue like syndrome as part of Long COVID.

Causes of ME/CFS

The causes of ME/CFS are multifactorial, involving a combination of genetic, environmental, and physiological factors. You will notice many similarities between ME/CFS and Long COVID that it is no wonder that the line begins to blur between these two conditions.

1. **Viral Infections**

    - Many people report the onset of ME/CFS following a viral infection. Common viruses linked to ME/CFS include Epstein-Barr virus (EBV), human herpesvirus 6 (HHV-6), enteroviruses, and cytomegalovirus (CMV).

    - **Long COVID**: Recent research suggests that post-viral syndromes, like Long COVID, can share similarities with

ME/CFS, leading to chronic fatigue and other overlapping symptoms.

2. **Immune Dysfunction**
    - ME/CFS patients often show signs of immune system abnormalities, including chronic inflammation, low-grade fevers, and fluctuations in immune markers.
    - There may be an overactive or dysfunctional immune response that leads to ongoing inflammation or an inability to regulate the body's response to infections or environmental triggers.
3. **Mitochondrial Dysfunction**
    - Mitochondria, the energy-producing structures in cells, may not function properly in people with ME/CFS, leading to a lack of energy production and severe fatigue.
    - Impaired mitochondrial function could explain the hallmark feature of post-exertional malaise (PEM), where even mild physical or mental exertion leads to a significant worsening of symptoms.
4. **Dysautonomia**
    - Many ME/CFS patients have autonomic nervous system dysfunction (dysautonomia), which affects heart rate, blood pressure, and digestion. Conditions like Postural Orthostatic Tachycardia Syndrome (POTS) are commonly seen in ME/CFS patients.
    - This dysregulation of the autonomic nervous system can cause symptoms such as lightheadedness, dizziness, and rapid heartbeat, especially upon standing.

5. **Gut Dysbiosis**

    - Alterations in the gut microbiome, including bacterial imbalances, are thought to contribute to ME/CFS. Abnormal gut flora may lead to increased intestinal permeability ("leaky gut"), allowing toxins to enter the bloodstream and trigger immune responses.

    - Gut-brain axis dysregulation may also affect energy levels and cognitive function in ME/CFS patients.

6. **Hormonal Imbalances**

    - Hypothalamic-pituitary-adrenal (HPA) axis dysfunction has been noted in ME/CFS patients, leading to abnormal levels of cortisol and other stress-related hormones.

    - This may contribute to fatigue, poor stress tolerance, and sleep disturbances seen in ME/CFS.

7. **Genetic Susceptibility**

    - Some individuals may have a genetic predisposition to developing ME/CFS, with certain genes involved in immune regulation, metabolism, and neurological function playing a role.

Symptoms of ME/CFS

- **Unrelenting fatigue**: Profound exhaustion not relieved by rest.

- **Post-exertional malaise (PEM)**: A significant worsening of symptoms following physical or mental exertion.

- **Cognitive issues**: Often referred to as "brain fog," involving problems with memory, focus, and processing information.

- **Sleep disturbances**: Unrefreshing sleep, insomnia, or sleep disorders.

- **Muscle and joint pain**: Widespread muscle pain, stiffness, and joint discomfort without swelling.
- **Headaches**: Chronic headaches or migraines.
- **Sensitivity to light, sound, or chemicals**: Increased sensitivity to environmental stimuli.

Symptom Management with Medications

Since ME/CFS presents a broad range of symptoms, treatment often involves a multi-faceted approach.

1. Pain Relief

Many ME/CFS patients experience chronic pain, including muscle pain, joint pain, and headaches. The following medications can help alleviate these symptoms:

- **Over-the-Counter (OTC)** Pain Relievers: Medications such as acetaminophen (*Tylenol*) and nonsteroidal anti-inflammatory drugs (NSAIDs) like *ibuprofen* (Advil, Motrin) and naproxen (Aleve) can offer relief from mild to moderate pain.
- **Prescription Pain Relievers:** For more severe pain, doctors may prescribe medications such as tramadol (Ultram) or low-dose tricyclic antidepressants like amitriptyline (Elavil), which can also help improve sleep quality.

2. Sleep Disorders

Sleep disturbances are common in ME/CFS, inducing various disorders such as difficulty falling asleep, staying asleep, or experiencing restorative sleep. Medications that may help include:

- **Sleep Aids:** OTC options like diphenhydramine (Benadryl) or prescription medications such as zolpidem (Ambien), eszopiclone (Lunesta), or low-dose antidepressants (*e.g.,* amitriptyline or trazodone) can be employed to improve sleep.

- **Melatonin:** A natural supplement that can help regulate the sleep-wake cycle and improve sleep quality.

3. Cognitive Symptoms

Cognitive dysfunction—often referred to as "*brain fog*"—is a significant symptom of ME/CFS. While no specific medication is approved for treating cognitive issues in ME/CFS, some patients find relief with:

- **Stimulants:** Medications like modafinil (*Provigil*) or methylphenidate (*Ritalin*) may be prescribed to help improve alertness and concentration. If used, I suggest short-term only.

- **Cognitive Enhancers:** Certain medications like donepezil (Aricept), which is typically used to treat *Alzheimer's* disease, have been used off-label to address cognitive symptoms in ME/CFS.

4. Orthostatic Intolerance

Orthostatic intolerance is a condition where standing up causes dizziness and lightheadedness. Orthostatic intolerance doesn't automatically mean that it is POTS. It is prevalent in ME/CFS patients. See POTS above for medications to treat this symptom.

5. Depression and Anxiety

Mental health conditions like depression and anxiety often accompany ME/CFS. Treating these conditions can improve overall well-being and quality of life. Common medications include:

- **Antidepressants:** Selective Serotonin Reuptake Inhibitors (SSRIs) like fluoxetine (Prozac) and sertraline (Zoloft), or serotonin-norepinephrine reuptake inhibitors (SNRIs) like duloxetine (Cymbalta) and venlafaxine (Effexor).

- **Anti-Anxiety Medications:** Benzodiazepines such as lorazepam (Ativan) or alprazolam (Xanax) can be used for short-term relief of anxiety symptoms.

Heart Rate Variability and Its Role in Managing Long COVID

Heart Rate Variability (HRV) is a robust, non-invasive measure of ANS function. It quantifies the variation in time between consecutive heartbeats, providing insight into the balance between the sympathetic (fight or flight) and parasympathetic (rest and digest) branches of the ANS. In recent years, HRV has gained attention for its potential role in monitoring and managing different health conditions, including Long COVID—a post-acute sequela of SARS-CoV-2 infection characterized by persistent symptoms lasting for weeks or months beyond the initial illness.

HRV is typically quantified using an electrocardiogram (ECG) or wearable devices with photoplethysmography (PPG) sensors. The data is analyzed to produce various metrics, including:

1. **Time-domain measures** include the standard deviation of all normal-to-normal intervals (**SDNN**) and the Root Mean Square of Successive Differences (**RMSSD**). **Takeaway point:** low numbers are alarming.

2. **Frequency-domain measures** include Low-Frequency (LF) and High-Frequency (HF) components corresponding to different autonomic regulation aspects.

We want a trend over 1-2 weeks rather than one number. Higher HRV is generally related to better cardiovascular fitness and a robust ability to adapt to stress, whereas lower HRV is linked to stress, fatigue, and poor health outcomes.

HRV and Long COVID

Long COVID encompasses a range of symptoms such as fatigue, brain fog, shortness of breath, and autonomic dysfunction. Many of these symptoms can be traced back to dysregulation of the ANS, making HRV a valuable tool for both evaluating and managing this condition.

Monitoring Autonomic Dysfunction

Patients with Long COVID often exhibit signs of autonomic dysfunction, including *Postural Orthostatic Tachycardia Syndrome* (POTS) and other forms of dysautonomia. Regular HRV monitoring can help detect these issues early, allowing timely intervention. Key indicators to watch for include:

- **Reduced overall HRV:** It indicates increased sympathetic dominance or decreased parasympathetic activity.
- **Altered LF/HF ratio:** Suggests an imbalance in autonomic control, a marker of stress or autonomic dysfunction.

HRV can guide personalized treatment strategies for Long COVID by providing real-time feedback on how interventions affect autonomic balance. All HRV is determined from the same data: the R-R or N-N time in milliseconds. The way the data is processed determines all of the HRV parameters.

Practical Applications

To incorporate HRV into the management of Long COVID, consider the following steps:

1. Decide what HRV parameter you will use and stick to it since we want to compare apples to apples, not apples to oranges.
    a. Decide which parameter your device uses, RMSSD or SDANN, as these are the more common ones, but make sure you always use the same device or software, as the

parameters are not interchangeable. The *Apple iWatch*, OORA ring, *Whoop* band, and polar chest straps can all be used. Pick something you will keep on, and it will be comfortable.

b. The gold standard is calculated from an ECG, but you can also use a light-based sensor.

c. Don't focus on any one HRV number. We are after trends over a few days to a few weeks.

2. Baseline Assessment: Establish a baseline with an initial HRV measurement. It can be done using a wearable device over a period of several days to capture typical daily fluctuations.

2. Regular Monitoring: Implement daily or weekly HRV evaluation to track changes over time. Pay attention to trends rather than single readings, as numerous factors, including sleep, stress, and illness, can influence HRV.

3. Adjust Interventions: Use HRV data to tailor interventions. For example, if HRV decreases following an increase in exercise intensity, consider reducing the intensity or duration until HRV improves.

4. Patient Education: Learn about the significance of HRV and how lifestyle factors such as sleep, nutrition, hydration, and stress management can influence their readings and overall well-being.

5. Multidisciplinary Approach: Collaborate with healthcare providers across disciplines to create a comprehensive management plan incorporating HRV monitoring. It could include primary care physicians, cardiologists, neurologists, physiotherapists, and cognitive health professionals.

Stellate Ganglion Block and Long COVID

Understanding Stellate Ganglion Block (SGB)

The stellate ganglion is a collection of nerves located in the neck, part of the sympathetic nervous system, which regulates many involuntary body functions. An SGB involves the injection of a local anesthetic around these nerves to block their activity temporarily. Is the Stellate Ganglion Block (SGB) only for taste and smell? No, it works to correct the dysautonomia.

How SGB Works

SGB is traditionally used to treat conditions such as chronic pain, Complex Regional Pain Syndrome (CRPS), and Post-Traumatic Stress Disorder (PTSD). The rationale behind its use in Long COVID is based on its ability to reset or modulate the sympathetic nervous system, potentially alleviating symptoms associated with autonomic dysfunction and inflammation.

Procedure

The SGB procedure is usually conducted in an outpatient setting by a trained specialist, such as an anesthesiologist or pain management physician. I perform this procedure under live ultrasound guidance, using an ultrasound visible needle, no steroids, and injecting both the C6 level and the C4 level. Only one side gets done at a time. You cannot block both left and right sides at the same time because it will create a surgical emergency where both sides of your vocal cords can close up so no air passes through. Any doctor who tells you it is safe for both sides simultaneously is not performing an actual stellate ganglion procedure.

Here is an overview of what the procedure involves:

1. **Preparation**: The patient is positioned, usually lying on their back with their neck slightly extended. Monitoring equipment is attached to track vital signs during the procedure.

2. **Ultrasound or Fluoroscopy Guidance**: To ensure precision, the physician utilizes ultrasound or fluoroscopy to locate the stellate ganglion accurately. I still prefer ultrasound guidance over fluoroscopy, where you can see arteries, veins, nerves, and muscles. Fluoroscopy only shows bone, and the area has essential structures.

3. **Injection**: A local anesthetic—such as bupivacaine, ropivacaine, or lidocaine—is injected around the stellate ganglion. The procedure typically takes about 15 minutes.

4. **Observation**: After the injection, the patient is monitored for any immediate side effects and to evaluate the initial efficacy of the block.

After the block is complete, you must see Horner's syndrome on the blocked side, which includes:

- A droopy eye, mainly the upper lid
- Redness on the white of the eye, the sclera
- A small pupil – I prefer to see a 2 mm or more difference, with the blocked side being smaller
    - Change in temperature on the blocked side by about 1 degree
    - The stuffy nose on the side blocked
    - Redness or flushing on the side blocked

Hoarseness or lump in the throat implies that you have blocked the recurrent laryngeal nerve and does NOT indicate that you have received an excellent sympathetic nervous system tract block.

I have treated thousands of patients with the stellate ganglion procedure. I have learned over these many procedures that what you put in is not as important as where you put it.

Stellate Ganglion Dominance

Similar to how we have a dominant hand, your body appears to select one side, right or left, to use more often to send sympathetic nervous system messages to the brain and body. In my experience, I have found that about:

- 80% are right dominant
- 10% are left dominant
- 10% are non-dominant

For this reason, we usually start on the right side.

Potential Benefits for Long COVID

Research into the use of SGB for Long COVID is in the early stages, but some promising results have been witnessed:

- **Symptom Relief:** Patients receiving SGB have reported improved symptoms such as fatigue, brain fog, and autonomic dysfunction. The exact mechanism is not entirely understood, but it is believed that modulating the sympathetic nervous system may reduce systemic inflammation and improve neural regulation.

Reduced Inflammation: SGB may help reduce the inflammatory response associated with Long COVID, potentially alleviating various symptoms associated with chronic inflammation.

  - natural killer cell activity reduction
  - reduction in levels of inflammatory cytokines such as IL-1, IL-4, IL-6, IL-8, and TNF-α

  - increase of anti-inflammatory cytokine IL-10 and calcitonin gene-related peptide (CGRP)
  - regulate endothelial dysfunction
  - regulate microcirculation
  - regulate coagulopathy
  - reduction of neurogenic pulmonary edema
  - pulmonary arterial hypertension reduction
  - reduction of pathological positive feedback loops

- **Autonomic Regulation:** Many Long COVID patients suffer from dysautonomia, in which the ANS fails to regulate heart rate, BP, and other functions properly. SGB might help restore regular autonomic operation.

Symptom relief specifics

- parosmia/dysgeusia
- anosmia/ageusia/ +/- hyposmia
- brain fog
- chronic fatigue
- exercise intolerance
- chest pain
- neuropathies in arms/hands/shoulders
- anxiety associated with PTSD or Long COVID
- PTSD
- Insomnia
- shortness of breath
- chronic cough
- chest pain

- joint pain
- tachycardia and palpitations
- diarrhea
- dizziness
- Headaches
- charges in the menstrual cycle
- rashes due to Long COVID
- fever

Risks and Considerations

- **Common Side Effects:** These can include temporary pain at the injection site, hoarseness, and difficulty swallowing. These side effects are usually temporary.
- **Serious Risks:** Though rare, complications such as bleeding, infection, nerve damage, or pneumothorax (collapsed lung) can occur. These risks underscore the importance of having the procedure performed by an experienced physician.
- **Horner's syndrome** – this is expected if you have an excellent sympathetic block
    - a droopy eyelid on the side of the injection
    - redness of the white of the eye
    - smaller pupil
    - stuffy nasal passage
    - change in skin temperature by about 1 degree Celsius
    - Flushing

Not all patients will respond to SGB uniformly. Some may experience significant relief, while others may have minimal or no improvement.

References:

1. Liu LD, Duricka DL. Stellate ganglion block reduces symptoms of Long COVID: A case series. J Neuroimmunol. 2022 Jan 15;362:577784. DOI:

   10.1016/j.jneuroim.2021.577784. Epub 2021 Dec 8. PMID: 34922127; PMCID: PMC8653406.

2. Khan MH, Kirkpatrick KP, Deng Y, Shah KB. Stellate Ganglion Block for Long COVID Symptom Management: A Case Report. Cureus. 2022 Dec 7;14(12):e32295. DOI: 10.7759/cureus.32295. PMID: 36628048; PMCID: PMC9822527.

3. Pearson L, Maina A, Compratt T, et al. (September 13, 2023) Stellate Ganglion Block Relieves Long COVID-19 Symptoms in 86% of Patients: A Retrospective Cohort Study. Cureus 15(9): e45161. DOI:10.7759/cureus.45161

4. Duricka D, Liu L. Reduction of Long COVID symptoms after stellate ganglion block: A retrospective chart review study. *Auton Neurosci.* 2024;103195.

   DOI:10.1016/j.autneu.2024.103195.

5. Mulvaney, S. W., Curtis, K. E., & Ibrahim, T. S. (2020, June 24). Comparison C6 Stellate Ganglion versus C6 and C4 Cervical Sympathetic Chain Blocks for Treatment of Posttraumatic Stress Disorder (PTSD): Analysis of 147 Patients. *Department of Military and Emergency Medicine, Uniformed Service University, USA*; *Regenerative Orthopedic and Sports Medicine, Maryland, USA.*

Vagus Nerve Dysfunction in Long COVID

Anatomy and Function

The vagus nerve—also known as cranial nerve X (10)—is the Longest cranial nerve, extending from the brainstem through the neck and thorax to the abdomen. It innervates significant organs, including the heart, lungs, and digestive tract. The vagus nerve plays a pivotal role in:

- **Cardiac Regulation:** Slowing the heart rate and promoting cardiovascular stability.
- **Digestive Function:** Stimulating peristalsis, secretion of digestive enzymes, and appetite regulation.
- **Immune Response:** Modulating inflammation through the "*cholinergic anti-inflammatory pathway*."
- **Mood and Stress Response:** It influences neurotransmitter release and stress resilience.

Vagus Nerve Dysfunction

Several mechanisms may underlie vagus nerve dysfunction in Long COVID:

1. **Direct Viral Impact**: SARS-CoV-2 may directly infect and damage the vagus nerve or its associated structures, impairing its function.

2. **Inflammatory Damage**: The inflammatory response to the virus can lead to cytokine release and subsequent neural inflammation, affecting vagal function.

3. **Immune-Mediated Damage:** Autoimmune responses triggered by the virus might target components of the vagus nerve.

4. **Oxidative Stress:** Persistent oxidative stress from ongoing inflammation can damage the vagus nerve and other neural tissues.

Symptoms Related to Vagus Nerve Dysfunction in Long COVID

Patients with Long COVID may experience a range of symptoms attributed to Vagus Nerve Dysfunction, including:

- **Cardiovascular Symptoms:** Palpitations, tachycardia, and hypotension.

- **Gastrointestinal Symptoms:** Nausea, vomiting, diarrhea, and abdominal pain.

- **Respiratory Symptoms:** Shortness of breath and difficulty breathing.

- **Neuropsychiatric Symptoms:** Anxiety, depression, brain fog, and fatigue.

- **General Symptoms:** Chronic pain and sleep disturbances.

Treating Vagus Nerve Dysfunction in Long COVID

- *Vagus Nerve Stimulation* (VNS) will be discussed in the next chapter.

- The EAT procedure (see *Epipharyngeal Abrasive Therapy* chapter).

Acetylcholinesterase Inhibitors

- Acetylcholinesterase inhibitors—such as **pyridostigmine**—can enhance cholinergic transmission by inhibiting the breakdown of acetylcholine, potentially improving vagus nerve function and reducing autonomic symptoms.

- **Huperzine A** is a supplement that has a similar mechanism.

Breathing Exercises

Deep breathing exercises, including diaphragmatic breathing and paced respiration, can stimulate the vagus nerve and promote relaxation. An easy breathing exercise is box breathing. It is named after the box-like pattern that you form.

1. Inhale for 4 seconds
2. Hold your breath for 4 seconds
3. Exhale for 4 seconds
4. Hold for 4 seconds
5. Repeat

If you cannot do it using four seconds, do three or fewer; just keep all 4 times the same. Do what you can.

Others

There are several ways to stimulate the vagus nerve, including humming, singing, yoga, tai chi, and massage therapy, which can all help you relax. These practices integrate physical movement, breathing exercises, and mindfulness, which can collectively improve vagal function and reduce symptoms of dysautonomia.

Vagus Nerve Stimulation

Near and dear to my heart, I have been using *transcutaneous Vagus Nerve Stimulation* (tVNS) for several years. It has been used to treat epilepsy, depression, migraines, and ulcerative colitis, and it shows promise for alleviating symptoms of Long COVID by enhancing vagal tone, reducing inflammation, and promoting healing, regeneration, and organ repair.

External ear vagus nerve stimulation is a non-invasive method that has shown promise in treating symptoms of Long COVID. This technique involves stimulating the auricular branch of the vagus nerve through the skin of the external ear, specifically targeting areas such as the tragus and cymba conchae.

Mechanism of Action

The vagus nerve is crucial in regulating autonomic functions such as heart rate, digestion, and inflammatory responses. By stimulating this nerve, tVNS can modulate the parasympathetic nervous system, which may help reduce inflammation and restore autonomic balance. This scenario is particularly relevant for Long COVID, where dysregulation of the ANS and persistent inflammation are thought to contribute to symptoms like fatigue, brain fog, and mood disturbances.

A study involving 24 female patients with Long COVID and continuous cognitive impairments underwent 10 days of tVNS treatment at home. The treatment sessions were conducted twice daily for 30 minutes each. Consequently, significant improvements were observed in cognitive functions, including attention, memory, and executive function.

Furthermore, secondary outcomes showed reductions in anxiety, depression, fatigue, and sleep disturbances.

Another study noted improvements in a broader set of symptoms such as fatigue, brain fog, widespread pain, and post-exertional malaise in Long COVID patients receiving tVNS. The study highlighted that many patients reported significant symptom relief, suggesting the potential of tVNS as a therapeutic modality for Long COVID.

Device and Treatment Protocol

The tVNS treatment involves the use of a device designed specifically for home use. Patients applied an electrode to the left ear tragus, delivering micro-pulses with a pulse width of 250 μs (microseconds) and a frequency of 25 Hz. Treatment personalization was based on individual sensitivity thresholds, ensuring that patients experienced a comfortable tingling sensation during the sessions.

Where Do I Place the Ear Clips?

Luckily for us, it is easy to stimulate the vagus nerve on the ear's surface. The simplest way to accomplish this is at the tragus of the ear. The idea is to stimulate the vagus nerve through the area surrounding the external ear opening called the meatus. The tragus is an ideal spot. Alternatively, you can use the cymba concha or the concha cavum. However, getting a clip to stay on in those areas is more complicated. It is also less comfortable than the tragus. Do NOT stimulate the ear lobe despite many YouTube videos and entries on Google suggesting that.

The vagus nerve is involved in 66%-80% of people with Long COVID. With imaging, it was shown thickened. The parasympathetic tone is lower than in those without Long COVID. Part of the autonomic dysfunction can be treated with this. This stimulation can be accomplished using an inexpensive TENS unit like the TENS 7000.

Please only stimulate one ear at a time. Remember that you must use two electrodes to complete the circuit. We recommend placing both electrodes on one ear. If you cannot, you can put one pad on the neck or upper back area with a pad instead. Please note that stimulation won't work with just one lead/electrode. Do not jam the clip into the external ear/auditory canal.

With low-intensity stimulation, it is likely safe to use both ears. However, the left ear is less likely to cause bradycardia or slowing of your heart. Limit stimulation to 30 minutes until you know how the stimulation impacts you. Check heart rate during right ear stimulation because it can potentially cause bradycardia.

You will need a unit to set the milliamps (mA), pulse width, and frequency. Some units have selectable *"programs* "and are preprogrammed for specific action setups only. Those are not good for what we want to do here. Those units are for *Electric Muscle Stimulation* (EMS) even though they call themselves TENS unit. There are also dedicated vagus nerve stimulators available.

> *Do NOT use if you have a pacemaker or defibrillator, are pregnant, or have a sick heart.*

Starting TENS parameters

Regular or continuous mode; do not use burst, EMS, or any other mode.

Use the left ear. The left ear spares the heart, so it is the safest ear to use. Using the right ear is also likely safe if the intensity is low.

- Frequency 25Hz (range 15-30 Hz)
- Pulse width 250 microseconds
- Intensity on TENS 7000: between 1-3.
- Once a day for 30 days.

Tips and Tricks

- The easiest way is to use a double-contact ear clip.
- If you use 2 single contact clips, ensure one lead clip is on the tragus.

- If you don't feel any tingling, try wetting the ear areas, including the tragus, with some tap water or saline eye drops.
- You can change the placement location for the lead, NOT on the tragus.
- You can switch the leads and change red to black and black to red.
- You can try a different clip type. I personally prefer the soft silicon black ones to the metal plate ones.

If you are not seeing ANY response or recovery after 30 days, do the following:

- Change to the right ear. Or switch back and forth. Monitor heart rate with right ear use.
- Switch the location of the ear to another (any part of the "inny" part of the ear, like the cymba concha or concha areas).
- Do the vagus nerve stim 2x/day, once in am, like 8 or 9 am, and once at pm, like at bedtime.
- Change frequency between 20-30Hz daily by a few numbers, Like 21 one day, 27 another, 24 another. Keep the vagus nerve from anticipating.
- Nothing should hurt or be uncomfortable. Nothing should twitch. Turn it down if it is painful and the intensity is too high.
- While I like to feel the tingling for the first 10-15 seconds, sometimes you don't. It is ok. Make sure the contact from the clips is good, and you can also use conductive gel instead of wetting.

References:

1. Verbanck, P., Clarinval, A. M., Burton, F., Corazza, F., Nagant, C., & Cheron, G. (2021). Transcutaneous auricular vagus nerve stimulation (tVNS) can reverse the manifestations of the Long-COVID syndrome: A pilot study. *Journal of Neurophysiology & Movement Biomechanics, Université Libre de Bruxelles*. Received April 10, 2021; Accepted May 13, 2021; Published May 21, 2021.

2. European Pharmaceutical Review. (2021, November 4). Long-COVID symptoms improved with neuromodulation. Retrieved from

   https://www.europeanpharmaceuticalreview.com/news/158262/Long-COVID-symptoms-improved-with-neuromodulation/

3. Badran, B. W., Huffman, S. M., Dancy, M., Austelle, C. W., & 3 more. (n.d.). A pilot randomized controlled trial of supervised, at-home, self-administered transcutaneous auricular vagus nerve stimulation (taVNS) to manage Long COVID symptoms. *Preprint*.

   https://DOI.org/10.21203/rs.3.rs-1716096/v1

4. Acanfora D, Nolano M, Acanfora C, Colella C, Provitera V, Caporaso G, Rodolico GR, Bortone AS, Galasso G, Casucci G. Impaired Vagal Activity in Long-COVID-19 Patients. Viruses. 2022 May 13;14(5):1035. DOI: 10.3390/v14051035. PMID: 35632776; PMCID: PMC9147759.

5. Natelson, B. H., Blate, M., & Soto, T. (2023). Transcutaneous vagus nerve stimulation in the treatment of Long COVID-chronic fatigue syndrome. *Archives of Clinical and Biomedical Research*, 7(2), 89-98.

   https://DOI.org/10.26502/acbr.50170337

6. Özden, A. V., & Perçin, A. (n.d.). A promising method for post-COVID/Long-COVID syndrome: Noninvasive vagus nerve stimulation. *Bahçeşehir University* and *Iğdır University*. https://DOI.org/10.5281/zenodo.8198614

7. Dani M, Dirksen A, Taraborrelli P, Torocastro M, Panagopoulos D, Sutton R, Lim PB. Autonomic dysfunction in 'Long COVID': rationale, physiology and management strategies. Clin Med (Lond). 2021 Jan;21(1):e63-e67. DOI: 10.7861/clinmed.2020-0896. Epub 2020 Nov 26. PMID: 33243837; PMCID: PMC7850225.

Epipharyngeal Abrasive Therapy (EAT)

Epipharyngeal Abrasive Therapy (EAT)—also known as epipharyngeal swab therapy—involves using a cotton swab to abrade the mucosa of the epipharynx. This therapy is sometimes used in Japan for chronic epipharyngitis and other conditions involving inflammation of the nasopharyngeal area. While it sounds simple, please don't try to do this alone at home. We use a flexible endoscopic camera and apply the cotton-tipped swab to particular areas while rubbing the nasopharynx and opening the *Eustachian* tube. EAT might help alleviate symptoms, particularly chronic inflammation in the nasopharyngeal area. The theory behind this therapy is that it can reduce local inflammation, which may contribute to systemic symptoms experienced by patients with Long COVID.

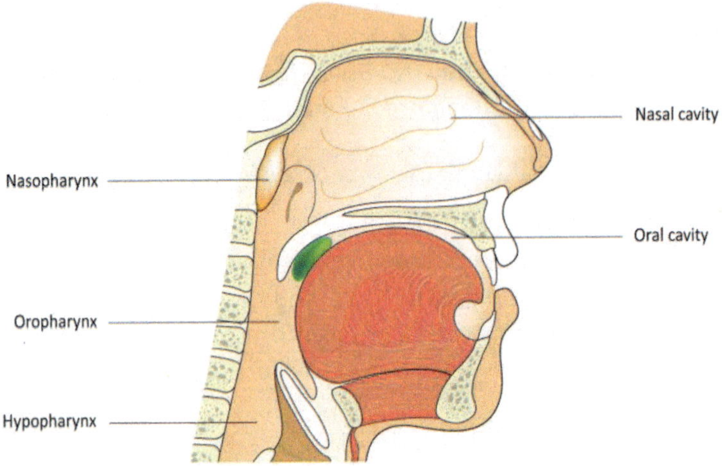

The "*epipharynx*" is not an actual anatomical structure. When coined, it refers to the area above and around the nasopharynx. Don't worry, and you won't gag during the procedure. We numb the area well with lidocaine. There are no injections; everything is applied topically.

Most patients with Long COVID also have chronic epipharyngitis, which is not always symptomatic, but many, if not all, people who suffer from Long COVID likely have it. It is responsible for causing many of the Long COVID symptoms. The immune system continues to respond as a residual response, causing neuroexcitatory molecules such as TNF-alpha, INF-delta, and IL-1 in the brain, resulting in low-level chronic inflammation. Symptoms like headaches, system-wide pain, fatigue, dizziness, throat pain, postnasal drip, and a chronic cough can also be witnessed. EAT has multiple effects:

- Direct stimulation of the vagus nerve endings
- decreased secretion of inflammatory cytokines
- suppression of inflammatory cell aggregation

What symptoms does EAT address?

- postnasal drip, runny nose
- irritated throat, headaches, and nasal irritation
- nasal congestion
- eustachian tube dysfunction, hearing loss, and tinnitus
- dizziness, vertigo, and lightheadedness
- hoarseness, voice changes
- cough, sore throat
- snoring, insomnia, and daytime sleepiness
- acid reflux, heartburn
- fatigue, brain fog, and depression

"I have seen visible and noticeable improvement with each EAT procedure. As the bleeding from the mucosa decreases, so do the symptoms. It is a great tool in the Long COVID treatment arsenal."

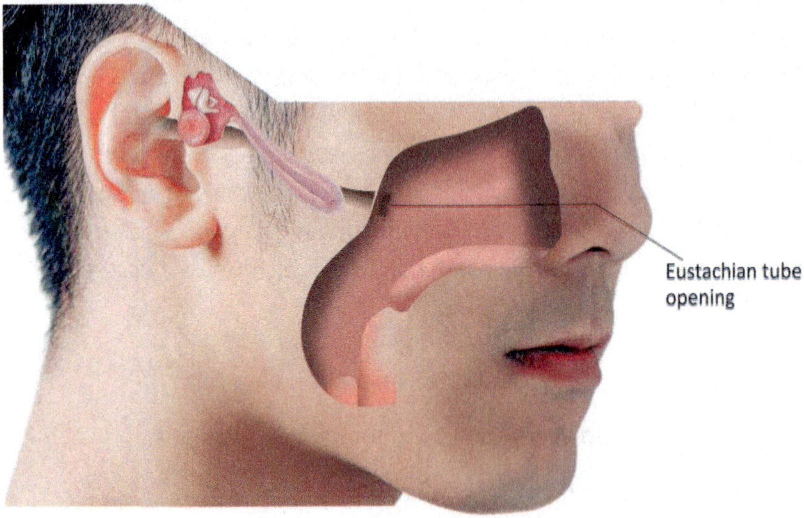

EAT Questionnaire

I use this questionnaire to determine if you would be a good candidate for this procedure and if you require more treatments. Essentially if you score 20 or more from this 0-50 range, you would qualify for the procedure. For repeat treatments, I use both a scope > 10 and the appearance of the epipharynx grade score.

Score: 0-50: ___________

- **Do I need an EAT Treatment?** If you score more than 10, you do.
- Can stop EAT treatments when score <= 10.

Symptoms	**Severity 0-5**
1. Postnasal drip symptoms (postnasal drip, runny nose, etc.)	0 1 2 3 4 5
2. Epipharyngeal irritation symptoms (irritated throat, headache, stiff neck, etc.)	0 1 2 3 4 5
3. Nose-related symptoms (runny nose, nasal congestion, nasal irritation, etc.)	0 1 2 3 4 5
4. Eustachian tube-related symptoms (ear fullness, hearing loss, tinnitus, etc.)	0 1 2 3 4 5
5. Vertigo-related symptoms (dizziness, light-headedness, etc.)	0 1 2 3 4 5
6. Voice-related symptoms (hoarseness, voice disturbances, etc.)	0 1 2 3 4 5

7. Laryngeal irritation symptoms (cough, sore throat, sore throat or discomfort, etc.)	0 1 2 3 4 5
8. Sleep apnea related symptoms (snoring, insomnia, daytime somnolence, etc.)	0 1 2 3 4 5
9. Gastrointestinal symptoms (acid reflux, heartburn, heavy stomach, etc.)	0 1 2 3 4 5
10. Autonomic symptoms (fatigue, chronic fatigue, brain fog, depressive symptoms, etc.)	0 1 2 3 4 5
Use value for each question: **0. No symptoms** **1. Slight symptoms/rarely bothers me.** **2. Mild symptoms, sometimes bothers me.** **3. Moderate symptom, almost always bothers me.** **4. Moderate-severe symptoms, always bothers me.** **5. Severe symptoms, intolerable.**	

References:

- Hirobumi Ito. Effect of Epipharyngeal Abrasive Therapy on Long COVID with Chronic Epipharyngitis. Sch J Oto. 8(5)-2022. SJO. MS.ID.000300. DOI: 10.32474/SJO.2022.08.000300 Sch J Oto Volume 8 - Issue 5

The HPA Axis and Long COVID

Hypothalamus – Pituitary – Adrenal (HPA) Axis

The HPA axis is an intricate network of interactions between the hypothalamus, pituitary gland, and adrenal glands. It plays a vital role in regulating:

- stress responses
- immune function
- digestion
- energy storage
- energy expenditure
- overall homeostasis

If the sympathetic nervous system is the heater and air conditioner, the pituitary is the wiring, and the hypothalamus is the thermostat.

Key Components of the HPA Axis

1. **Hypothalamus:** the hypothalamus is located in the brain and releases *Corticotropin-Releasing Hormone* (CRH) in response to stress.
2. **Pituitary Gland:** CRH stimulates the pituitary gland to *Secrete Adrenocorticotropic Hormone* (ACTH).

3. **Adrenal Glands:** ACTH triggers the adrenal glands, located atop the kidneys, to release cortisol, the body's primary stress hormone.

Function of the HPA Axis

The HPA axis controls the body's reaction to stress through a feedback loop:

- In response to stress, the hypothalamus releases CRH.
- CRH prompts the pituitary gland to release ACTH.
- ACTH stimulates the adrenal glands to create cortisol.
- Elevated cortisol levels help the body manage stress and signal the hypothalamus and pituitary to reduce CRH and ACTH production, maintaining balance.

HPA Axis Dysregulation and Long COVID

Emerging research recommends that Long COVID may involve dysregulation of the HPA axis. This dysregulation could contribute to multiple chronic symptoms experienced by Long COVID patients.

Possible Mechanisms of Dysregulation

1. **Chronic Stress Response:** The prolonged stress of a severe infection like COVID-19 can lead to an overactive HPA axis, resulting in consistently high cortisol levels. Over time, this can exhaust the system, leading to low cortisol levels and an impaired stress response.

2. **Immune System Interaction:** The HPA axis interacts closely with the immune system. Chronic inflammation from a prolonged immune response to COVID-19 could disrupt normal HPA axis function, leading to a feedback loop of stress and inflammation.

3. **Autonomic Nervous System (ANS) Involvement:** The ANS, which controls involuntary bodily functions, works alongside the HPA

axis. Dysautonomia—or dysfunction of the ANS—is common in Long COVID and may be associated with HPA axis dysregulation.

Symptoms Linked to HPA Axis Dysfunction

The symptoms of HPA axis dysregulation in Long COVID patients may include:

- **Fatigue:** Chronic cortisol imbalance can lead to feelings of severe and continuous fatigue.
- **Sleep Disturbances:** Dysregulation can influence sleep patterns, leading to insomnia or unrefreshing sleep.
- **Cognitive Impairment:** Often referred to as *"brain fog,"* this impairment includes challenges with concentration, memory, and mental clarity.
- **Mood Disorders:** Anxiety, depression, and mood swings can result from chronic stress and cortisol imbalance.
- **Pain and Inflammation:** Altered cortisol levels can impact the body's inflammatory response, contributing to muscle and joint pain.

Several ongoing studies are exploring the role of the HPA axis in Long COVID. These studies offer the following insights:

1. **Cortisol Levels in Long COVID Patients:** Some studies have observed that Long COVID patients exhibit altered cortisol levels—either elevated due to chronic stress or reduced due to HPA axis exhaustion. These findings suggest a potential link between cortisol imbalance and Long COVID symptoms.

2. **Stress and Immune System Interaction:** Research has highlighted the bidirectional relationship between stress and immune function, where prolonged inflammation due to COVID-19 can exacerbate stress responses and vice versa. This interaction can perpetuate HPA axis dysregulation.

3. **Potential Therapeutic Interventions:** Understanding HPA axis involvement in Long COVID opens up new avenues for treatment. Interventions that aim to restore HPA axis balance are being explored, including stress management techniques, lifestyle modifications, and specific medications.

Managing HPA Axis Dysfunction in Long COVID

Addressing HPA axis dysfunction involves a multifaceted approach:

1. **Stress Management:** Techniques such as mindfulness, meditation, and yoga can help reduce stress and promote HPA axis balance.

2. **Regular Physical Activity:** Moderate exercise can improve HPA axis function and reduce stress. However, it should be approached cautiously in Long COVID patients to prevent post-exertional malaise.

3. **Healthy Sleep Hygiene:** Improving sleep quality through persistent sleep schedules, a comfortable sleep ecosystem, and relaxation techniques can support HPA axis regulation.

4. **Balanced Nutrition:** A nutrient-rich diet can support overall health and HPA axis function. Avoiding stimulants like caffeine and maintaining stable blood sugar levels are also important.

5. **Medical Interventions:** In some cases, medications or supplements that support adrenal function and hormone balance may be prescribed. A healthcare provider should always manage these. I can help with this.

6. **Treat the dysautonomia** – this is the part that I can help you with.

Hormonal Menstrual Abnormalities

Understanding Testosterone and Estrogen

Testosterone and estrogen are vital hormones that play significant roles in the body. While commonly linked to male and female characteristics, both hormones are present in all individuals, albeit in different amounts.

Testosterone is primarily produced in the testes in males and smaller amounts in the ovaries and adrenal glands in females. It is responsible for developing male secondary sexual characteristics, such as increased muscle mass, body hair, and a deeper voice. Besides, testosterone plays a role in mood regulation, libido, and overall energy levels.

Estrogen, on the other hand, is primarily produced in the ovaries in females and smaller quantities in the testes and adrenal glands in males. It is crucial for developing female secondary sexual characteristics, such as breast development and the regulation of the menstrual cycle. Moreover, estrogen also contributes to bone health, cardiovascular function, and cognitive abilities.

Hormonal Dysregulation in Long COVID

The exact mechanisms by which Long COVID affects hormonal balance are still being studied. However, there are several plausible pathways through which the SARS-CoV-2 virus could disrupt endocrine function:

1. **Direct Viral Effects:** The virus may directly invade endocrine glands, leading to altered hormone production. For instance, ACE2

receptors, which the virus uses to enter cells in endocrine tissues, suggest that these glands could be targets for viral infection.

2. **Immune Response and Inflammation:** Long COVID is associated with a prolonged inflammatory response. Chronic inflammation can impact the Hypothalamic-Pituitary-Gonadal (HPG) axis, which regulates the production of sex hormones. Inflammation can disrupt this axis, leading to imbalances in hormone levels.

3. **Stress Response:** The psychological and physiological stress of dealing with a chronic illness like Long COVID can also affect hormonal balance. The Hypothalamic-Pituitary-Adrenal (HPA) axis, which controls the body's response to stress, can influence the production of sex hormones. Chronic stress can lead to elevated cortisol levels, which may suppress the production of testosterone and estrogen.

Testosterone in Long COVID

In individuals with Long COVID, disruptions in testosterone levels have been reported. Low testosterone levels can lead to various symptoms, including fatigue, depression, reduced libido, and muscle weakness. These symptoms can overlap with common Long COVID manifestations, making it challenging to disentangle the specific contributions of hormonal imbalances.

Potential Mechanisms

- **Inflammation:** Chronic inflammation can suppress the production of testosterone. Cytokines, which are elevated in inflammatory states, can inhibit gonadotropin-releasing hormone (GnRH) secretion, reducing the stimulation of testosterone production.

- **Direct Testicular Damage:** Evidence shows that SARS-CoV-2 can infect the testes, potentially leading to direct damage and impaired testosterone production.

Estrogen in Long COVID

In addition, estrogen dysregulation has also been observed in individuals with Long COVID. Estrogen is vital for maintaining menstrual health, and imbalances can lead to menstrual abnormalities.

Potential Mechanisms

- **Ovarian Dysfunction:** Similar to testosterone, the ovaries may be affected directly by the virus or the prolonged inflammatory response. It can lead to altered estrogen production.

- **HPA Axis Disruption:** Chronic stress and elevated cortisol levels can disrupt the HPG axis, impacting estrogen and menstrual cycle regulation.

Menstrual Abnormalities in Long COVID

Many patients with Long COVID have reported variations in their menstrual cycles, including irregular periods, heavier or lighter bleeding, and increased *Premenstrual Syndrome* (PMS) symptoms. These menstrual abnormalities can significantly impact the quality of life and may indicate underlying hormonal imbalances.

Common Menstrual Abnormalities

- **Amenorrhea:** The absence of menstrual periods for three or more months can occur due to disrupted estrogen production.

- **Oligomenorrhea:** Infrequent menstrual periods—occurring more than 35 days apart—can result from hormonal imbalances.

- **Menorrhagia:** Heavy menstrual bleeding can be caused by an imbalance in estrogen and progesterone levels, leading to excessive endometrial growth and shedding.

Clinical Management and Future Directions

Addressing hormonal imbalances and menstrual abnormalities in Long COVID necessitates a multidisciplinary approach. Caregivers should consider the following strategies:

1. **Hormonal Assessments:** Regular monitoring of hormone levels, including testosterone and estrogen, can help identify imbalances and guide treatment.

2. **Anti-inflammatory Therapies:** Managing chronic inflammation through medications and lifestyle changes may help restore hormonal balance.

3. **Stress Management:** Techniques such as mindfulness, therapy, and stress-reducing activities can support the HPA axis and improve hormonal regulation.

4. **Gynecological Care:** Patients experiencing menstrual abnormalities should seek specialized care to address these issues and receive appropriate interventions.

5. **Treat the dysautonomia:** This is the part that I will help you with.

Vitamin D, Phosphorus, and Calcium

Vitamin D deficiency is common in Long COVID. While Vitamin D can be made in our skin, there is not enough made to be useful. Therefore, it is still considered an essential nutrient that we must get from food or supplements. Having a severe Vitamin D deficiency can cause rickets or brittle bones.

Vitamin D comes in 2 natural forms

1) Vitamin D2 (**ergocalciferol**) from plants, mushrooms, and yeasts

2) Vitamin D3 **(cholecalciferol, 7-dehydrocholesterol)** comes from fish oil, egg yolk, tuna, salmon, and skin UV-B exposure; 3x more potent than vitamin D2).

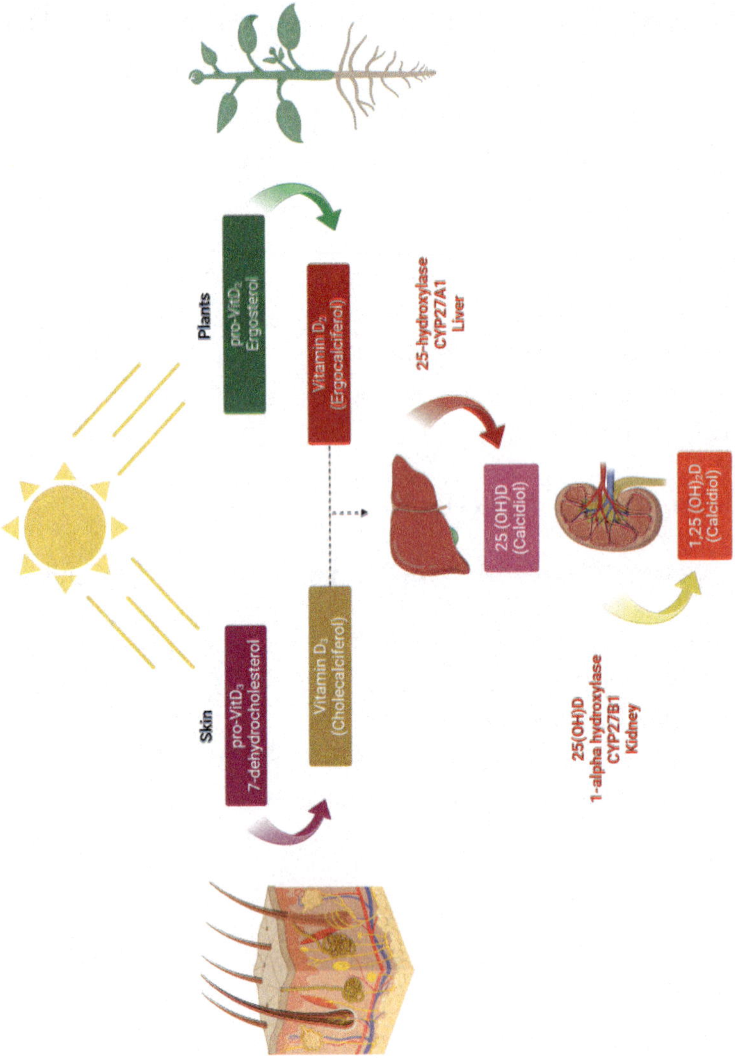

Vitamin D (**cholecalciferol**) is also synthesized in our skin from exposure to UV-B light.

Both are fat soluble, but D3 is more effective at raising your levels.

Vitamin D blood levels

- Levels of 50 nmol/L (20 ng/mL) or above are adequate for most people for bone.
- Levels below 30 nmol/L (12 ng/mL) are too low and might weaken your bones.
- Levels above 125 nmol/L (50 ng/mL) are too high.

What Causes Vitamin D deficiency?

- Kidney or liver failure, which prevents the body from adequately processing vitamin D.
- limited sunlight exposure
- reduced capacity of the skin to synthesize vitamin D
- Darker skin pigment
- Malnutrition
- Certain medications
    - Laxatives
    - Steroids (such as prednisone)
    - Cholesterol-lowering drugs (such as cholestyramine and colestipol)
    - Seizure-preventing drugs (such as phenobarbital and phenytoin)
    - Rifampin (a tuberculosis drug)
    - Orlistat (a weight-loss drug)
- Certain types of cancer, such as lymphoma
- A family history of vitamin D deficiency or childhood rickets

What are the early symptoms of vitamin D deficiency?

- Most will be asymptomatic!
- Fatigue

- Not sleeping well
- Bone pain or achiness
- Depression or feelings of sadness
- Hair loss
- Muscle weakness
- Loss of appetite
- Getting sick more easily
- Pale skin

What are the chronic and extreme symptoms of prolonged vitamin D deficiency?

- softening and weakening of bones called rickets, in children, osteomalacia in adults.
- sudden cardiac death (SCD)
- myocardial infarction (MI)
- stroke and cardiovascular events (CE)
- death due to heart failure
- fatal infections and all-cause mortality.

How do Vitamin D, magnesium, calcium, and phosphorus, all interact?

- **Vitamin D stimulates intestinal calcium and phosphorus absorption.**
- Need vitamin D to absorb calcium.
- Need magnesium to activate vitamin D in kidneys.
- Magnesium intake can reduce calcium absorption.
- Calcium can increase magnesium excretion.
- Phosphates bind to magnesium and don't get absorbed.
- Low circulating magnesium can impair vitamin D metabolism (breakdown), leading to increased calcium absorption (more active vit D in circulation).

- an existing magnesium deficiency may result in a vitamin D level that does not increase as much as expected in response to vitamin D supplementation.

How do we activate Vitamin D?

- **It is biologically inactive after being ingested or made in the skin**
- It is hydroxylated in the liver into **calcidiol** or **calcifediol** (25-hydroxyvitaminD).
- It is catalyzed by a 2nd hydroxylation in the kidney into calcitriol (100x more active than other forms) – 1,25-dihidroxyvitaminD
- Circulates in the blood bound to vitamin D binding protein and albumin as **cholecaciferol** and **ergocalciferol** and this is what we measure from a blood test.

Symptoms of hypercalcemia (High calcium in blood)

- Digestive symptoms, such as nausea or vomiting, poor appetite, or constipation
- Increased thirst or more frequent urination, due to changes in the kidneys
- Muscle weakness or twitches
- Changes in how your brain works, such as feeling tired or fatigued or confused
- Bone pain and fragile bones that break more easily

GASTROINTESTINAL

- Pancreatitis
- Peptic ulcer disease

KIDNEY

- Calcium deposits in the kidney (nephrocalcinosis) that cause poor kidney function
- Dehydration
- High blood pressure

- Kidney failure
- Kidney stones

PSYCHOLOGICAL

- Depression
- Difficulty concentrating or thinking

SKELETAL

- Bone cysts
- Fractures
- Osteoporosis

Chronic kidney disease usually required vitamin D supplementation due to low 1,25 (OH) vitamin D

Hypercalcemia & Vitamin D

- Most commonly from parathyroid gland overactivation
- Can be caused by decreased kidney excretion of calcium
- Cancer – with bone erosion
- Sarcoidosis

What does PTH do? – goal is to <u>increase</u> blood calcium levels

- Causes bone to release calcium, bone remodeling
- Inhibits reabsorption of phosphate in kidney
- Increases resorption of calcium in kidneys
- Increases activation of vitamin D to 1,25 vitD – stimulates calcium absorption from intestines.

Parathyroid hormone is stimulated by:

- Decreased serum [Ca^{2+}].
- Mild decreases in serum [Mg^{2+}].
- An increase in serum phosphate (increased phosphate causes it to complex with serum calcium, forming calcium phosphate, which

reduces stimulation of Ca-sensitive receptors (CaSr) that do not sense calcium phosphate, triggering an increase in PTH).

- **Epinephrine (Adrenaline)**
- **Histamine**

Hypocalcemia (low calcium in blood) symptoms

- **Acute** hypocalcemia can result in severe symptoms requiring hospitalization, whereas patients who **gradually develop hypocalcemia** are more likely to be asymptomatic.
- paresthesias
- muscle spasms
- muscle cramps
- tetany
- circumoral numbness
- seizures
- laryngospasm
- neuromuscular irritability
- cognitive impairment
- personality disturbances
- prolonged QT intervals
- electrocardiographic changes that mimic myocardial infarction
- heart failure

Vitamin D Supplementation

1. Bone Health and Calcium Homeostasis

- **Promotes Calcium Absorption**: Vitamin D enhances the absorption of calcium and phosphorus in the gut, which are crucial for maintaining strong bones and teeth.

- **Prevents Rickets and Osteomalacia**: In children, vitamin D deficiency can lead to rickets, a condition characterized by soft, weak bones. In adults, a similar condition known as osteomalacia can occur. Supplementation helps prevent and treat these disorders.

- **Osteoporosis Prevention**: Vitamin D, along with calcium, helps in preventing osteoporosis, especially in postmenopausal women and older adults. It aids in maintaining bone density and reducing the risk of fractures.

2. Immune Function

- **Boosts Immune Response**: Vitamin D plays a vital role in modulating the innate and adaptive immune systems. It enhances the pathogen-fighting abilities of monocytes and macrophages, key cells of the immune system, and decreases inflammation.

- **Reduction of Respiratory Infections**: Several studies suggest that vitamin D supplementation may reduce the risk of acute respiratory tract infections. This has gained attention during the COVID-19 pandemic, where vitamin D's role in immune modulation was explored for potential protective effects against severe COVID-19 outcomes.

3. Cardiovascular Health

- **Blood Pressure Regulation**: Vitamin D may play a role in reducing high blood pressure (hypertension), which is a risk factor for cardiovascular diseases.

- **Heart Disease**: Some evidence suggests that vitamin D deficiency is linked to an increased risk of heart disease, but research on supplementation has shown mixed results. Adequate vitamin D levels may help reduce the risk of cardiovascular problems, including heart attacks and strokes.

4. Mood and Mental Health

- **Depression and Anxiety**: Low levels of vitamin D have been linked to mood disorders such as depression and anxiety. Vitamin D receptors are present in many brain areas associated with mood regulation, suggesting that supplementation may help improve symptoms of depression, particularly in people who are deficient.

- **Cognitive Function**: Vitamin D may have a protective role against cognitive decline in older adults, though more research is needed to confirm this.

5. Diabetes and Metabolic Health

- **Type 2 Diabetes**: Vitamin D may improve insulin sensitivity and help regulate blood sugar levels. Some studies suggest that low levels of vitamin D are associated with an increased risk of developing type 2 diabetes.

- **Metabolic Syndrome**: Adequate vitamin D levels are linked to a lower risk of metabolic syndrome, a cluster of conditions (high blood pressure, high blood sugar, abnormal cholesterol levels, and excess body fat around the waist) that increase the risk for heart disease and type 2 diabetes.

6. Autoimmune Diseases

- **Multiple Sclerosis (MS)**: Vitamin D deficiency has been linked to an increased risk of developing MS, and supplementation may reduce the severity and frequency of relapses.

- **Rheumatoid Arthritis and Lupus**: Vitamin D has anti-inflammatory effects, and low levels have been associated with the development of autoimmune diseases like rheumatoid arthritis and lupus. Supplementation may help modulate immune responses in these conditions.

7. Cancer Prevention

- **Colorectal, Breast, and Prostate Cancer**: Some research suggests that higher levels of vitamin D may reduce the risk of certain cancers, particularly colorectal cancer. The role of vitamin D in cancer prevention may be related to its ability to regulate cell growth, differentiation, and apoptosis (programmed cell death).

8. Muscle Function and Strength

- **Muscle Weakness**: Vitamin D is essential for muscle strength, and low levels are associated with muscle weakness and an increased risk of falls, especially in the elderly.

- **Sarcopenia**: Adequate vitamin D intake may help prevent sarcopenia (age-related muscle loss) and improve physical performance.

9. Pregnancy and Fetal Development

- **Bone Health for the Fetus**: Pregnant women need adequate vitamin D to support fetal bone development and calcium metabolism.

- **Prevention of Pregnancy Complications**: Vitamin D deficiency has been associated with a higher risk of preeclampsia, gestational diabetes, and low birth weight.

References:

- Aghajafari, F., et al. (2013). **Association between maternal serum 25-hydroxyvitamin D level and pregnancy and neonatal outcomes**. *BMJ*, 346, f1169.

- Visser, M., et al. (2003). **Low vitamin D and muscle strength**. *Journal of Clinical Endocrinology & Metabolism*, 88(12), 5766-5772.

- Garland, C. F., et al. (2006). **The role of vitamin D in cancer prevention**. *American Journal of Public Health*, 96(2), 252-261.

- Pittas, A. G., et al. (2007). **Vitamin D and calcium intake in relation to type 2 diabetes in women**. *Diabetes Care*, 30(3), 650- Munger, K. L., et al. (2006). **Vitamin D intake and incidence of multiple sclerosis**. *Neurology*, 66(5), 772-778.656.

- Mozos, I., & Marginean, O. (2015). **Links between vitamin D deficiency and cardiovascular diseases**. *BioMed Research International*, 2015.

- Anglin, R. E., et al. (2013). **Vitamin D deficiency and depression in adults**: *British Journal of Psychiatry*, 202(2), 100-107.

- Martineau, A. R., et al. (2017). **Vitamin D supplementation to prevent acute respiratory tract infections**: *BMJ*, 356, i6583.

- Grant, W. B., et al. (2020). **Evidence that vitamin D supplementation could reduce the risk of influenza and COVID-19 infections and deaths**. *Nutrients*, 12(4), 988.

- Holick, M. F. (2006). **Vitamin D deficiency**. *New England Journal of Medicine*, 357(3), 266-281.

Histamine

Histamine is a biogenic amine involved in various physiological processes such as immune response, gastric acid secretion, and neurotransmission. Mast cells are one of the white blood cells. It is stored in mast cells and basophils and released during immune reactions. Histamine is made from an essential amino acid, histidine. Essential means that we cannot manufacture it in our bodies or in enough quantities to be helpful. Therefore, all of the histamine comes from histidine that we eat or drink. Histamine and mast cells are the third possible cause of Long COVID. There is more to histamine that causes hives and itching.

Histamine Receptors

Histamine actually works through four types of receptors. Everyone knows the 2 that we have medications for the H1 and H2 blockers.

- **H1 Receptors**: These are involved in allergic responses, vasodilation, bronchoconstriction, and neurotransmission.
- **H2 Receptors**: Regulate gastric acid secretion and play a role in immune modulation.
- **H3 Receptors**: These receptors are involved in neurotransmission and modulating the release of other neurotransmitters.
- **H4 Receptors**: Play a role in immune response and inflammation.

What does histamine do?

1. Immune Response

- **Allergic Reactions:** Histamine is released from mast cells and basophils during allergic reactions. It binds to histamine receptors (primarily H1 receptors) on various cells, leading to multiple symptoms like itching, swelling, redness, and bronchoconstriction.

- **Inflammation:** Histamine contributes to the inflammatory response by increasing the permeability of blood vessels, allowing white blood cells and other immune proteins to access infected or damaged tissues more quickly.

2. Gastric Secretion

- **Stomach Acid Production:** Histamine stimulates gastric acid secretion in the stomach. It binds to H2 receptors on parietal cells in the stomach lining, promoting the production and release of hydrochloric acid, which aids in digestion.

3. Neurotransmitter Functions

- **Brain Activity:** Histamine acts as a neurotransmitter in the brain, which regulates wakefulness, arousal, and appetite. It binds to H1 and H3 receptors in the central nervous system.

4. Regulation of Physiological Functions

- **Vasodilation:** Histamine causes the dilation of blood vessels, which can lead to decreased BP. This vasodilatory effect is essential in regulating blood flow to different tissues.

- **Smooth Muscle Contraction:** Histamine can cause smooth muscle contraction, primarily in the lungs and gastrointestinal tract, influencing respiratory and digestive functions.

5. Role in Homeostasis

- **Temperature Regulation:** Histamine is involved in regulating body temperature and energy balance.

- **Circadian Rhythm:** Histamine levels in the brain fluctuate throughout the day, playing a role in regulating the sleep-wake cycle.

Methylation's part in Histamine Metabolism

Methylation plays a crucial role in the **metabolism of histamine** in the body, particularly in the breakdown and regulation of histamine levels in tissues, including the brain. The process involves adding a **methyl group (CH_3)** to histamine, which is primarily catalyzed by the enzyme **Histamine N-Methyltransferase (HNMT)**. This enzyme is key to maintaining balanced histamine levels, preventing histamine excess, which can lead to a range of physiological and pathological effects.

Key Steps in Histamine Methylation:

1. **Histamine Production**
    - Histamine is produced from the amino acid **histidine** through the action of the enzyme **histidine decarboxylase**. It functions as a neurotransmitter and plays a role in immune responses, gastric acid secretion, and inflammatory reactions.
2. **Histamine Breakdown by Methylation**
    - The enzyme **Histamine N-Methyltransferase (HNMT)** methylates histamine by adding a methyl group to its imidazole ring.
    - This methylation process converts histamine into **N-methylhistamine**, which is an inactive metabolite.
    - The **methyl group** is donated by **S-adenosylmethionine (SAMe)**, which is the major methyl donor in the body. SAMe is synthesized from methionine through the methionine cycle, which itself relies on sufficient levels of vitamins such as **B12** and **folate**.

- **N-methylhistamine** is further broken down into **N-methylimidazole acetic acid** by **monoamine oxidase B (MAO-B)**, completing histamine degradation.

Methylation in Different Tissues

- **Histamine N-Methyltransferase (HNMT)** is primarily active in the **brain**, **liver**, **kidneys**, and **bronchial epithelium**, where it plays a key role in inactivating histamine to regulate its effects on the nervous and immune systems.
- In other tissues, such as the **gut**, **diamine oxidase (DAO)** is the main enzyme responsible for breaking down histamine. DAO degrades histamine through a different pathway, converting histamine into **imidazole acetaldehyde** rather than methylating it.

Consequences of Impaired Methylation

1. **Histamine Excess (Histamine Intolerance)**
    - When methylation capacity is impaired due to reduced **HNMT activity** or insufficient **SAMe**, histamine is not efficiently broken down, leading to **elevated histamine levels**. This can result in symptoms of **histamine intolerance**, such as:
        - Flushing
        - Headaches or migraines
        - Itching and hives
        - Gastrointestinal symptoms (diarrhea, bloating)
        - Respiratory issues (nasal congestion, bronchospasms)
        - Neurological symptoms (irritability, anxiety)

2. **Genetic Variations (Polymorphisms)**
    - Certain **polymorphisms** in the **HNMT gene**, such as the **Thr105Ile** polymorphism, can reduce the enzyme's activity, impairing histamine breakdown. This has been associated with conditions like **Parkinson's Disease** and potentially **schizophrenia**, as histamine dysregulation in the brain can affect neurotransmission and inflammation.
    - Reduced methylation capacity, whether from genetic factors or nutrient deficiencies (e.g., **B12, folate, methionine**), can exacerbate histamine-related issues.
3. **Methylation and Neuroinflammation**
    - In the brain, histamine acts as a neurotransmitter, influencing wakefulness, cognition, and immune responses. Impaired histamine methylation in the central nervous system could contribute to neuroinflammatory processes, which are implicated in neurodegenerative and psychiatric disorders like **Parkinson's Disease**, **multiple sclerosis**, and **schizophrenia**.

Supporting Histamine Metabolism through Methylation

To support efficient histamine breakdown via methylation, it is essential to ensure proper function of the **methylation cycle**. Key factors include:

- **Adequate levels of vitamins B6, B12, and folate**, which are necessary for the synthesis of SAMe.
- **Methionine** and **choline-rich foods** can also support methylation by providing essential building blocks for SAMe synthesis.
- **Methylfolate** (methylated folate) supplements may be beneficial for individuals with methylation defects, such as those with MTHFR gene polymorphisms, to enhance methylation capacity.

References:

1. Patel RH, Mohiuddin SS. Biochemistry, Histamine. [Updated 2023 May 1]. In: StatPearls [Internet]. Treasure Island (FL): StatPearls Publishing; 2024 Jan-. Available from: https://www.ncbi.nlm.nih.gov/books/NBK557790/

2. Thangam, E. B., Jemima, E. A., Singh, H., Baig, M. S., Khan, M., Mathias, C. B., Church, M. K., & Saluja, R. (2018). The role of histamine and histamine receptors in mast cell-mediated allergy and inflammation: The hunt for new therapeutic targets. *Frontiers in Immunology, 9,* 1873. https://doi.org/10.3389/fimmu.2018.01873

3. Carthy, E., & Ellender, T. (2021). Histamine, neuroinflammation and neurodevelopment: A review. *Frontiers in Neuroscience, 15,* 680214. https://doi.org/10.3389/fnins.2021.680214

4. Maintz, L., & Novak, N. (2007). Histamine and histamine intolerance. *The American Journal of Clinical Nutrition, 85*(5), 1185–1196.

5. Yang, X., et al. (2015). Association of Histamine N-Methyltransferase Thr105Ile Polymorphism with Parkinson's Disease and Schizophrenia in Han Chinese: A Case-Control Study. *PLOS ONE, 10*(3), e0119692. https://doi.org/10.1371/journal.pone.0119692

6. Ohtsu, H. (2010). Histamine and Histamine Receptors in Health and Disease. *Springer Science & Business Media.*

Diamine Oxidase (DAO) Enzyme

DAO is an enzyme found in the body, primarily in small intestine and kidneys. Its primary function is to break down histamine, a compound naturally produced by the body and found in certain foods. Moreover, immune cells also release histamine during allergic reactions and inflammation. Individuals with histamine intolerance may experience symptoms due to either excessive histamine intake from foods (such as aged cheeses, fermented foods, and alcohol) or impaired DAO activity in the gut. DAO supplementation aims to improve the body's ability to metabolize histamine, thereby reducing symptoms like headaches, digestive issues, skin problems, and respiratory difficulties.

- **Function**: DAO helps to degrade histamine into its byproducts, which are then removed from the body. This enzymatic activity is vital in maintaining histamine balance in the body.
- **Role in Health**: In individuals with sufficient DAO activity, histamine from ingested food or generated in the body is effectively broken down, preventing the accumulation of excess histamine in the bloodstream.
- **Implications in Health Conditions**: Reduced DAO activity or deficiency can lead to histamine intolerance or sensitivity. Histamine intolerance occurs when the body cannot properly metabolize histamine, leading to headaches, digestive issues, skin problems, and respiratory difficulties.

Copper's Role in DAO Function

Copper plays a crucial role in the enzymatic activity of DAO. DAO is a copper-containing enzyme, and adequate copper levels are required for its proper functioning. Copper acts as a cofactor in DAO's catalytic process, enabling the breakdown of histamine. Therefore, a deficiency in copper may impair DAO activity, leading to reduced histamine degradation and heightened symptoms of histamine intolerance.

Copper Deficiency and DAO Dysfunction

Copper deficiency can arise from poor dietary intake, malabsorption, or conditions that impair copper metabolism. When copper levels are low, DAO activity may be compromised, leading to reduced histamine metabolism. This can contribute to or exacerbate histamine intolerance in affected individuals. Conversely, ensuring adequate copper levels can help support optimal DAO function and alleviate symptoms associated with excess histamine.

How to use DAO supplements?

- DAO supplements are typically taken orally before meals or along with meals. The DAO enzyme works in the digestive tract to break down histamine from ingested food before it can be absorbed into the bloodstream. It is best to take DAO with catalase enzyme to reduce the hydrogen peroxide, a byproduct of histamine metabolism. The hydrogen peroxide can inactivate the DAO enzyme if not neutralized.

References:

1. Jochum C. Histamine Intolerance: Symptoms, Diagnosis, and Beyond. Nutrients. 2024 Apr 19;16(8):1219. doi: 10.3390/nu16081219. PMID: 38674909; PMCID: PMC11054089.

2. Hrubisko M, Danis R, Huorka M, Wawruch M. Histamine Intolerance-The More We Know the Less We Know. A Review. Nutrients. 2021 Jun 29;13(7):2228. doi: 10.3390/nu13072228. PMID: 34209583; PMCID: PMC8308327.

3. Legleiter LR, Spears JW. Plasma diamine oxidase: a biomarker of copper deficiency in the bovine. J Anim Sci. 2007 Sep;85(9):2198-204. doi: 10.2527/jas.2006-841. Epub 2007 May 25. PMID: 17526663.

Mast Cells

Mast cells are white blood cells crucial to the body's immune response. They are found in tissues throughout the body, especially at sites of potential injury, such as the skin, lungs, and digestive tract. Mast cells release histamine and other mediators in response to various triggers, including allergens, infections, and stress.

Remember that mast cells have much more than histamine inside them. Besides histamine, many other bioactive chemicals and mediators include heparin, cytokines, growth factors, proteases (break down protein), and many more.

Mast cells are immune cells that play a key role in allergic reactions, inflammation, and host defense. They contain a variety of **granules** inside them, which store preformed inflammatory and immune mediators. Upon activation, mast cells undergo a process called **degranulation**, during which they release these stored substances into the surrounding tissues. This release triggers inflammatory and immune responses.

Key Mediators Released by Mast Cells Upon Degranulation:

1. **Histamine**
    - One of the most well-known mediators, histamine causes **vasodilation**, **increased vascular permeability**, and **smooth muscle contraction**. This results in classic allergic symptoms such as itching, swelling, redness, and bronchoconstriction.

2. **Proteases**

    - **Tryptase** and **chymase** are enzymes stored in mast cells that degrade proteins in the extracellular matrix. These proteases contribute to tissue remodeling, inflammation, and the recruitment of other immune cells.

3. **Heparin**

    - Heparin is an **anticoagulant** that prevents blood clotting. It helps to maintain blood flow in areas of inflammation but can also contribute to bleeding in certain pathological conditions.

4. **Cytokines and Chemokines**

    - Mast cells release **pro-inflammatory cytokines** such as **TNF-α**, **IL-4**, **IL-6**, **IL-13**, and **GM-CSF**, which modulate the immune response by activating other immune cells like neutrophils, eosinophils, and lymphocytes.

    - **Chemokines**, like **CCL2 (MCP-1)** and **CXCL8 (IL-8)**, recruit other immune cells to the site of inflammation, especially during allergic reactions and infections.

5. **Lipid Mediators** (Synthesized upon degranulation)

    - Upon activation, mast cells rapidly synthesize and release lipid mediators such as:

        - **Prostaglandins** (e.g., **Prostaglandin D2 (PGD2)**): Promote vasodilation, bronchoconstriction, and leukocyte recruitment.

        - **Leukotrienes** (e.g., **Leukotriene C4 (LTC4)**): Strongly induce **bronchoconstriction** and increase **vascular permeability**, which can lead to asthma and allergic rhinitis symptoms.

- **Platelet-activating factor (PAF)**: Increases vascular permeability and plays a role in bronchoconstriction and inflammation.

6. **Serotonin**

   - In some species (e.g., rodents), mast cells release **serotonin**, which acts as a neurotransmitter and vasoconstrictor, contributing to vascular changes and inflammation.

7. **Growth Factors**

   - Mast cells can release **VEGF (vascular endothelial growth factor)**, which promotes the formation of new blood vessels (angiogenesis) and enhances vascular permeability.

Effects of Mast Cell Degranulation

- **Allergic Reactions**: Mast cell degranulation is a central feature of **type I hypersensitivity reactions**, which include **anaphylaxis, asthma, urticaria (hives)**, and **hay fever**. The release of histamine and other mediators leads to rapid onset symptoms like itching, swelling, airway constriction, and hypotension in severe cases.

- **Inflammation and Tissue Repair**: Mast cells also play a role in wound healing and tissue repair. The release of proteases and cytokines can stimulate tissue remodeling, recruit other immune cells, and contribute to chronic inflammation if over-activated.

- **Infection Defense**: Mast cells release their contents in response to pathogens, helping to recruit immune cells like neutrophils and macrophages to the site of infection.

References:

1. Thangam, E. B., Jemima, E. A., Singh, H., Baig, M. S., Khan, M., Mathias, C. B., Church, M. K., & Saluja, R. (2018). The Role of Histamine and Histamine Receptors in Mast Cell-Mediated Allergy and Inflammation: The Hunt for New Therapeutic Targets. *Frontiers in Immunology, 9,* 1873. https://doi.org/10.3389/fimmu.2018.01873

2. da Silva, E. Z. M., Jamur, M. C., & Oliver, C. (2014). Mast cell function: A new vision of an old cell. *Journal of Histochemistry and Cytochemistry, 62*(10), 698-738. https://doi.org/10.1369/0022155414545334

Mast Cell Activation Syndrome (MCAS)

The inappropriate activation and release of mediators from mast cells characterize MCAS. It can lead to a wide range of symptoms, often mimicking allergic reactions, but without an apparent external trigger.

Symptoms of MCAS

Symptoms of MCAS can vary widely and impact several organ systems, including:

- **Skin**: Urticaria (hives), flushing, itching.
- **Ear, Nose, Throat (ENT)**: throat tightening sensation, runny nose, sinus irritation
- **Gastrointestinal:** Nausea, vomiting, diarrhea, abdominal pain and cramping, and bloating.
- **Respiratory:** Wheezing, shortness of breath, and nasal congestion.
- **Cardiovascular:** Tachycardia, hypotension, dizziness, palpitations, pre-syncope (feeling like you are about to pass out).
- **Neurological:** Headaches, brain fog, and fatigue.

Diagnosing MCAS is difficult due to its extensive range of symptoms and lack of specific biomarkers. Diagnosis typically involves:

- A comprehensive patient history
- Symptom evaluation
- Laboratory tests measuring levels of tryptase, histamine, and prostaglandin D2

- Response to treatment with mast cell stabilizers and antihistamines

Histamine, MCAS, and Long COVID

1. **Immune Dysregulation:** SARS-CoV-2 infection can lead to prolonged immune activation and dysregulation, which may cause inappropriate mast cell activation.
2. **Persistent Inflammation:** Chronic inflammation observed in Long COVID can promote mast cell activation and histamine release.
3. **Viral Persistence**: Ongoing presence of viral particles may continuously trigger mast cells.
4. **Autoimmunity:** SARS-CoV-2 may trigger autoantibodies that target mast cells or their receptors, leading to continuous activation.

Treating Histamine Intolerance and MCAS

Antihistamines

- **H1 Antihistamines:** Cetirizine, loratadine, and diphenhydramine can help alleviate symptoms like itching, hives, and nasal congestion.
- **H2 Antihistamines**: Famotidine and ranitidine can decrease gastric acid secretion and help manage gastrointestinal symptoms.
- **Quercetin**
- Stinging nettle
- Vitamin D
- Luteolin
- EGCG
- Butterbur

Mast Cell Stabilizers

- **Cromolyn Sodium:** This medication can stabilize mast cells and prevent the release of mediators, helping to reduce symptoms. Can be sprayed as a nasal spray or taken orally.
- **Ketotifen** used to be available orally commercially in US, but now it must be compounded to be consumed orally.
- **Vitamin C**
- **Turmeric:** curcumin has anti-inflammatory effects.
- **Ginger:** Has anti-inflammatory and antioxidant properties.
- **Butterbur:** Can minimize histamine release and help manage allergic symptoms.
- **Luteolin**
- **Apigenin**
- **Quercetin**
- **Fisetin**
- **Kaempferol**
- **EGCG**
- **Silymarin**
- **Resveratrol**
- **Honokiol (magnolia bank extract)**
- **Curcumin**
- **Threonine**
- **Ellagic acid**

Leukotriene Receptor Antagonists

Montelukast: It can block leukotrienes, inflammatory mediators released by mast cells, and help reduce respiratory and allergic symptoms.

Nutritional and Dietary Interventions

Dietary modifications can help control histamine intolerance and reduce mast cell activation.

Low-Histamine Diet

A low-histamine diet avoids foods high in histamine or those that trigger histamine release. Typical high-histamine foods include:

- Aged cheeses, fermented foods, and alcoholic beverages.
- Processed meats, certain fish (*e.g.,* tuna, mackerel), and shellfish.
- Tomatoes, spinach, eggplants, and avocados.

Nutritional Supplements

- **Vitamin C**: An antioxidant that can help reduce histamine levels.
- **Vitamin B6**: Plays a role in histamine breakdown and helps manage symptoms.
- **Quercetin**: A bioflavonoid with mast cell stabilizing and anti-inflammatory properties.

Stress Management

Chronic stress can exacerbate mast cell activation. Techniques such as mindfulness, meditation, yoga, and deep-breathing exercises can help manage stress and reduce symptoms.

Environmental Modifications

Detecting and avoiding environmental triggers such as allergens, strong odors, and extreme temperatures can help manage symptoms.

References:

1. Sumantri, Stevent; Rengganis, Iris. Immunological dysfunction and mast cell activation syndrome in Long COVID. Asia Pacific Allergy 13(1):p 50-53, March 2023. | DOI: 10.5415/apallergy.0000000000000022

2. Weinstock LB, Brook JB, Walters AS, Goris A, Afrin LB, Molderings GJ. Mast cell activation symptoms are prevalent in Long-COVID. *Int J Infect Dis*. 2021;112:217-226. DOI:10.1016/j.ijid.2021.09.043.

3. Malone RW, Tisdall P, Fremont-Smith P, Liu Y, et al. COVID-19: Famotidine, Histamine, Mast Cells, and Mechanisms. Preprint. DOI:10.21203/rs.3.rs-30934/v3.

4. Finn DF, Walsh JJ. Twenty-first-century mast cell stabilizers. Br J Pharmacol. 2013 Sep;170(1):23-37. DOI:

   10.1111/bph.12138. PMID: 23441583; PMCID:

   PMC3764846.

5. Nutrition Issues in Gastroenterology, Series #199. (2020). Mast Cell Activation Syndrome – What it Is and Isn't.

6. Kettner L, Seitl I, Fischer L. Toward Oral Supplementation of Diamine Oxidase for the Treatment of Histamine Intolerance. Nutrients. 2022 Jun 24;14(13):2621. DOI:

   10.3390/nu14132621. PMID: 35807806; PMCID:

   PMC9268349.

Probiotics

Certain strains of probiotics can help reduce histamine levels by either promoting gut health or degrading histamine, thus providing relief for individuals with histamine intolerance. Some probiotic strains are known to produce lower levels of histamine or may even support the breakdown of histamine in the gut, making them beneficial for people sensitive to histamine.

Low Histamine-Producing Probiotic Strains

1. **Bifidobacterium species**
   - **Bifidobacterium infantis**
   - **Bifidobacterium longum**
   - **Bifidobacterium breve**
   - **Bifidobacterium bifidum**
   - These strains do not produce histamine and may improve gut health, reduce inflammation, and support the degradation of histamine.

2. **Lactobacillus species**
   - **Lactobacillus plantarum**
     - Well-studied for its anti-inflammatory properties and ability to degrade biogenic amines like histamine.
   - **Lactobacillus rhamnosus**

        - This strain has been shown to support the intestinal barrier and does not contribute to histamine production. It is often recommended for individuals with histamine intolerance.
    - **Lactobacillus gasseri**
        - This strain is low in histamine production and can help modulate the immune response.

3. **Saccharomyces boulardii**
    - This probiotic yeast strain does not produce histamine and is useful for supporting gut health. It can help in reducing inflammation and preventing histamine-related symptoms.
4. **Streptococcus thermophilus**
    - Known for its role in dairy fermentation, this strain is considered safe for those with histamine intolerance as it does not produce histamine.

Mechanism and Benefits

- **Reduction in Histamine Levels**: These probiotics help by promoting a healthy gut environment, maintaining the integrity of the intestinal barrier, and supporting proper immune function. They do not release histamine themselves, and some may help in breaking down histamine through their enzymatic activity.

- **Anti-inflammatory Properties**: Probiotics such as **Lactobacillus plantarum** and **Bifidobacterium longum** exhibit anti-inflammatory effects, which can help mitigate histamine-related inflammatory responses.

- **Gut Microbiome Support**: By promoting the growth of beneficial bacteria and reducing the abundance of histamine-producing microbes (such as certain strains of **Escherichia coli**, **Enterococcus**, and **Lactobacillus reuteri**), these probiotics can help balance histamine levels in the body.

Avoid High Histamine-Producing Strains

While incorporating low-histamine probiotics, it's also important to avoid strains known for high histamine production, such as:

- **Lactobacillus casei**
- **Lactobacillus bulgaricus**
- **Lactobacillus helveticus**

These strains are more likely to produce histamine and may exacerbate symptoms in individuals with histamine intolerance.

Probiotics are live bacterium cultures that we want to populate our gut. Moreover, they can be beneficial and displace any pathologic species that have moved in. Look for live and active cultures on the label. Probiotics often come from fermented food products and products that use live cultures such as kefir, yogurt, sauerkraut, kombucha, kimchi, aged cheese, miso, natto, apple cider vinegar (If not pasteurized and raw), kvass.

Soil-based, **Bacillus** spore-forming bacteria are generally more resistant to harsh stomach acid conditions, high temperatures, and radiation. Furthermore, they have benefits similar to those of ***Lactobacillus*** and ***Bifidobacterium*** species but have a greater chance of surviving and colonizing the large intestine.

Other Treatments

- Collagen
- Bovine Colostrum
- Lactoferrin
- Metformin

References:

1. Lau RI, Su Q, Lau ISF, Ching JYL, Wong MCS, Lau LHS, Tun HM, Mok CKP, Chau SWH, Tse YK, Cheung CP, Li MKT, Yeung GTY, Cheong PK, Chan FKL, Ng SC. A synbiotic preparation (SIM01) for post-acute COVID-19 syndrome in Hong Kong (RECOVERY): a randomised, double-blind, placebo-controlled trial. Lancet Infect Dis. 2024 Mar;24(3):256-265. DOI: 10.1016/S1473-3099(23)00685-0. Epub 2023 Dec 7. PMID: 38071990.

2. Singh K, Rao A. Probiotics: A potential immunomodulator in COVID-19 infection management. Nutr Res. 2021 Mar;87:1-12. DOI: 10.1016/j.nutres.2020.12.014. Epub 2021 Feb 13. PMID: 33592454; PMCID: PMC7881295.

3. Marinoni, B., Rimondi, A., Bottaro, F., Ciafardini, C., Amoroso, C., Muià, M., Caridi, B., Noviello, D., Bandera, A., Gori, A., Mantero, M., Blasi, F., Ferrucci, R., Facciotti, F., Vecchi, M., & Caprioli, F. (2023). The Role of VSL#3® in the Treatment of Fatigue and Other Symptoms in Long COVID-19 Syndrome: a Randomized, Double-blind, Placebo-controlled Pilot Study (DELong#3). DOI:

4. https://DOI.org/10.1101/2023.06.28.23291986

5. Vinderola G, Sanders ME, Salminen S. The Concept of Postbiotics. Foods. 2022 Apr 8;11(8):1077. DOI: 10.3390/foods11081077. PMID: 35454664; PMCID: PMC9027423.

6. **Sanders, M. E., et al. (2019)**. Probiotics and prebiotics in dietetics practice. *Journal of the American Dietetic Association*, 119(2), 278-287. doi:10.1016/j.jand.2018.11.005

7. **Szczuko, M., et al. (2020)**. Probiotics and their role in managing histamine intolerance: A review. *Critical Reviews in Food Science and Nutrition*, 60(15), 2507-2521. doi:10.1080/10408398.2019.1641549

8. **Mizuno, C. S., et al. (2018)**. Probiotics and histamine intolerance: A review. *Frontiers in Nutrition*, 5, 52. doi:10.3389/fnut.2018.00052

9. Hill, C., Guarner, F., Reid, G., Gibson, G. R., Merenstein, D. J., Pot, B., ... & Sanders, M. E. (2014). *Expert consensus document: The International Scientific Association for Probiotics and Prebiotics consensus statement on the scope and appropriate use of the term probiotic.* Nature Reviews Gastroenterology & Hepatology, 11(8), 506-514.

10. Marco, M. L., & Tachon, S. (2013). *Environmental factors influencing the efficacy of probiotic bacteria.* Current Opinion in Biotechnology, 24(2), 207-213.

Bifidobacterium and Lactobacillus Species

11. **O'Hara, A. M., & Shanahan, F. (2006)**. The gut flora as a forgotten organ. *EMBO Reports*, 7(7), 688-693. doi:10.1038/sj.embor.7400738

12. **Feng, W., Wang, W., Wang, Y., et al. (2019)**. Probiotics and their metabolites attenuate intestinal inflammation and increase gut barrier function in a mouse model of ulcerative colitis. *Frontiers in Microbiology*, 10, 2124. doi:10.3389/fmicb.2019.02124

Lactobacillus plantarum

13. **Pereira, M. I., de Oliveira, J. A., da Costa, L. B., et al. (2018)**. Lactobacillus plantarum reduces systemic and intestinal inflammation in mice with experimental colitis. *Journal of Nutritional Biochemistry*, 59, 1-9. doi:10.1016/j.jnutbio.2018.05.013

14. **Wang, S., Xie, Z., Zhao, H., et al. (2020)**. Lactobacillus plantarum alleviates allergic inflammation by regulating the immune response in the intestines. *Molecular Immunology*, 123, 125-134. doi:10.1016/j.molimm.2020.06.023

Saccharomyces boulardii

15. **Kailasapathy, K., & Ruckmani, K. (2015)**. Probiotics and their potential health benefits. *Indian Journal of Medical Research*, 142(2), 150-158. doi:10.4103/0971-5916.176374

16. **Shornikova, A. V., Olesen, J., et al. (1997)**. The non-pathogenic yeast Saccharomyces boulardii in the treatment of antibiotic-

associated diarrhea in children. *Pediatric Infectious Disease Journal*, 16(7), 702-705. doi:10.1097/00006454-199707000-00014

Streptococcus thermophilus

17. **Mollestad, H. M., et al. (2017)**. The probiotic strain Streptococcus thermophilus ST10 increases gut microbiota diversity and supports immune function in mice. *Frontiers in Microbiology*, 8, 865. doi:10.3389/fmicb.2017.00865

Gut Dysbiosis in Long COVID

The Gut Microbiome

The gut microbiome contains trillions of microorganisms, including bacteria, viruses, fungi, and archaea, which reside in the gastrointestinal tract. This is normal. While discussing the gut microbiome, you have these neighborhoods all over your body. This complex ecosystem plays vital roles in digestion, immune modulation, and overall health. A balanced gut microbiome is critical in maintaining homeostasis and preventing disease.

Most of the gut microbiome is in the colon. While there are bacterial The colonies in the stomach and small bowel, are on orders of magnitude less than the colon.

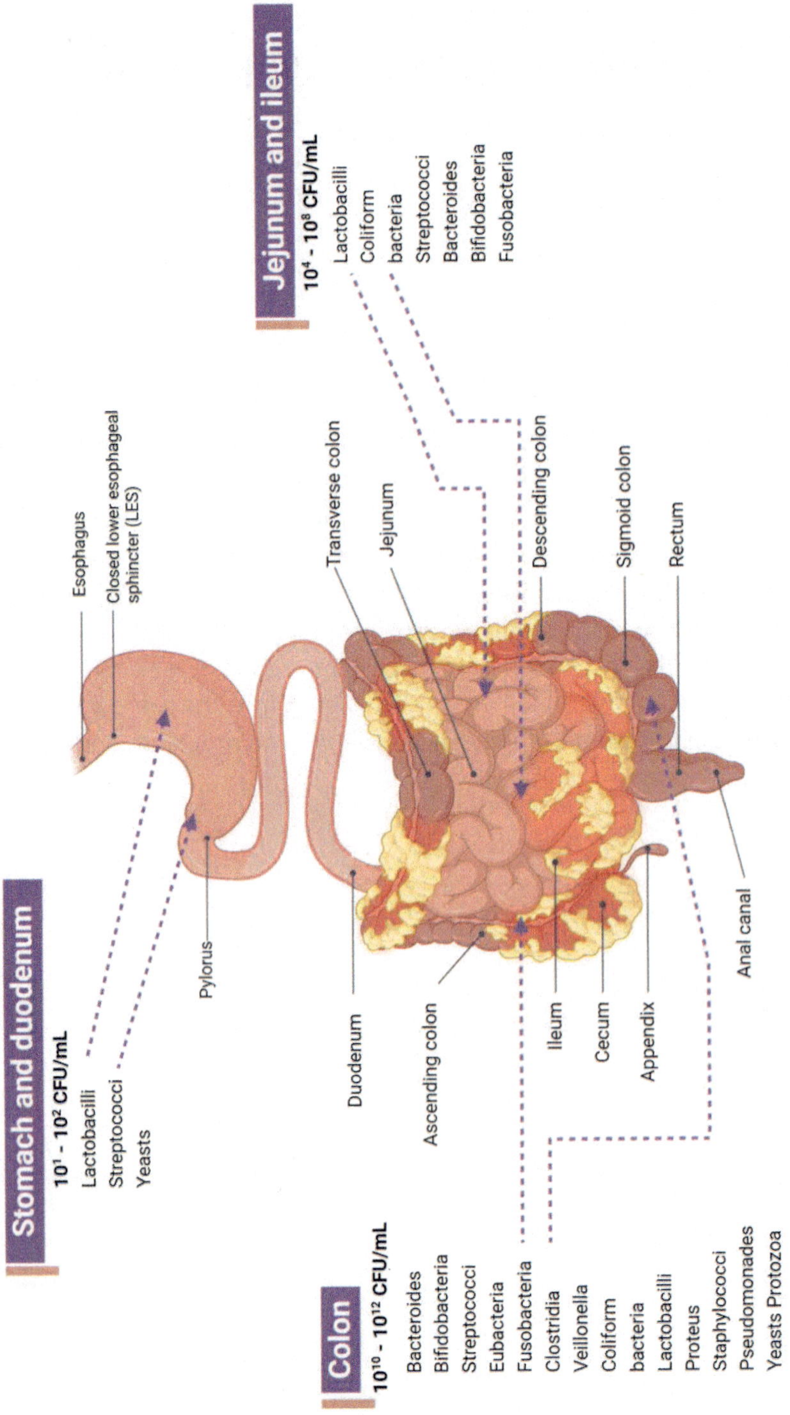
Stomach and duodenum
10^1 - 10^2 CFU/mL
Lactobacilli
Streptococci
Yeasts
Jejunum and ileum
10^4 - 10^8 CFU/mL
Lactobacilli
Coliform bacteria
Streptococci
Bacteroides
Bifidobacteria
Fusobacteria
Colon
10^{10} - 10^{12} CFU/mL
Bacteroides
Bifidobacteria
Streptococci
Eubacteria
Fusobacteria
Clostridia
Veillonella
Coliform bacteria
Lactobacilli
Proteus
Staphylococci
Pseudomonades
Yeasts Protozoa
Esophagus
Closed lower esophageal sphincter (LES)
Pylorus
Duodenum
Ascending colon
Transverse colon
Jejunum
Descending colon
Sigmoid colon
Rectum
Ileum
Cecum
Appendix
Anal canal

Dysbiosis and Health

Dysbiosis is a disruption of the helpful bacteria that live in our gut called our microbiome. Dysbiosis occurs from:

1. decreased microbial diversity
2. imbalance between beneficial and harmful microorganisms
3. reduction or elimination of certain species. In Long COVID, the two most involved ones are *Lactobacillus* and *Bifidobacterium*.

It can be caused by:

4. antibiotic use
5. poor diet, infections
6. chronic diseases
7. including inflammatory bowel disease
8. Irritable Bowel Syndrome (IBS)
9. metabolic disorders
10. Long COVID

Gut Dysbiosis in Long COVID

Recent studies have demonstrated that SARS-CoV-2 can directly impact the gut microbiome, leading to dysbiosis. Patients with Long COVID frequently report symptoms such as diarrhea, abdominal pain, and bloating, which may be associated with an altered gut microbiome. Furthermore, gut dysbiosis can aggravate systemic inflammation and immune dysregulation, potentially prolonging and intensifying Long COVID symptoms.

Gut-Organ Axis

- ### Gut-Brain Axis
    - The brain and gut talk to each other through the vagus nerve and neurotransmitters. Your gut and brain communicate through nerves, hormones, and immune signals. Thus, it can affect your mood, stress, and conditions like anxiety and depression.
    - Hormones such as **cortisol**, **serotonin**, and others are involved in the communication between the gut and brain.
    - Gut microbiota affects the production of neurotransmitters such as serotonin and dopamine, and disruptions here can impact mood and cognitive abilities.
- ### Gut-Liver Axis
    - The liver processes nutrients and toxins from the gut. It has substantial implications for liver health and conditions like fatty liver disease.
- ### Gut-Kidney Axis
    - Toxins from the gut can impact kidney function, influencing chronic kidney disease and overall kidney health.
- ### Gut-Heart Axis
    - Gut bacteria produce substances that can affect heart health. It is related to conditions like heart disease and high blood pressure.
- ### Gut-Lung Axis
    - How it works: Gut health affects lung immune responses and inflammation. It impacts respiratory conditions like asthma and COPD.

The gut and the microbiome strongly influence many organs. Disruptions here don't just remain in the gut.

What if the Colon is Surgically Removed?

People can survive a **total colectomy** (complete removal of the colon) because the **small intestine** can largely take over the function of absorbing nutrients, <u>even though the gut microbiome is affected</u>. Here's how survival and adaptation occur:

1. Nutrient Absorption

- **Small Intestine's Role**: The small intestine remains intact after a colectomy, and it is responsible for most nutrient absorption, including proteins, carbohydrates, fats, vitamins, and minerals. Thus, the body can still acquire most essential nutrients.

- **Adaptation**: The small intestine may adapt over time by increasing its absorptive capacity, a process called **intestinal adaptation**, which can help compensate for the loss of the colon's functions.

2. Water and Electrolyte Balance

- **Colon's Role**: The colon is mainly involved in absorbing water and electrolytes, and its removal can lead to issues with hydration and diarrhea initially.

- **Post-Surgery Management**: People often need to be vigilant about hydration and may need to modify their diets to avoid dehydration. Over time, the small intestine can adapt to absorb more water, but managing fluids through diet or medications is critical, particularly in the early recovery phase.

3. Stoma or J-Pouch

- **Ileostomy**: After a total colectomy, the end of the small intestine (the ileum) may be brought through an opening in the abdominal wall (stoma) to create an ileostomy. Waste is then collected in a bag outside the body. This allows the patient to live without a colon.

- **Ileal Pouch-Anal Anastomosis (J-Pouch)**: In some cases, surgeons create a J-pouch from the small intestine, which is connected to the anus, allowing waste to pass normally. This can help patients live without a stoma while maintaining some level of natural waste expulsion.

4. Impact on Gut Microbiome

- **Microbiome Changes**: The colon houses a large portion of the body's microbiome, which aids in digesting complex carbohydrates, producing vitamins (e.g., Vitamin K, certain B vitamins), and regulating immune function. Without a colon, a significant portion of these bacteria is lost.

- **Adaptation and Supplementation**: Some bacteria may recolonize the small intestine, but the overall diversity and function of the microbiome are reduced. Probiotic supplementation or dietary changes may be used to support digestive health, although the exact composition of the microbiome will not return to its original state.

5. Long-Term Consequences

- **Diarrhea and Short Bowel Syndrome**: Some patients may experience chronic diarrhea or **short bowel syndrome** (especially if parts of the small intestine were also removed), which can lead to malabsorption of nutrients and require careful dietary management or nutrient supplementation.

- **Dietary Adjustments**: After a colectomy, individuals often need to adopt a low-fiber diet and avoid foods that can cause blockages or increase stool output. Managing nutrient intake and hydration becomes essential.

6. Managing Life After Colectomy

- **Diet and Medications**: Patients may need a specialized diet (low-fiber, small frequent meals) and medications like **anti-diarrheal agents** or **electrolyte supplements**.
- **Lifestyle**: Regular monitoring of hydration and electrolyte levels is critical, and some may require intravenous fluids if oral intake is insufficient.

Malnutrition and Starvation

Some people are unable to eat much due to conditions like gastroparesis, nausea, vomiting, a persistent feeling of fullness, lack of appetite, abdominal bloating, or pain. But prolonged malnutrition and starvation go far beyond Long COVID—they cause extensive damage throughout the body. This issue is more than just a matter of diet or consulting a nutritionist. If you're consistently losing weight, your body is in a state of catabolism, where it's breaking down its own tissues and organs for survival. You must do whatever it takes to get enough calories, nutrients, and essential vitamins.

If your gut works, use it—even if you're not hungry. Remember, not eating is not an option—survival is the goal. If you can't eat enough, consider a feeding tube, which can be placed percutaneously by a gastroenterologist or surgeon and directly into your stomach. In extreme cases, short-term TPN (total parenteral nutrition) may be used when the gut is temporarily unusable, but it's not a long-term solution. Prolonged IV nutrition can lead to liver damage. High-calorie liquids can also be delivered directly through a feeding tube.

Restoring nutrition after prolonged starvation must be done gradually to avoid **refeeding syndrome**, a potentially life-threatening condition.

If you're not fully aware of the long-term effects of severe caloric restriction, let me explain:

1. Chronic inflammation

2. Severe oxidative stress
3. Loss of the body's ability to neutralize free radicals
4. Damage to vital organs like the liver, heart, and kidneys due to oxidative damage
5. Accelerated aging
6. Excessive autophagy
7. Excessive muscle breakdown
8. Severe mitochondrial dysfunction
9. Excessive fat breakdown, leading to lipid peroxidation, which can damage other organs, DNA, and more

This is why getting proper nutrition is essential for your body to repair and recover.

Refeeding syndrome

While I know you may be eager to gain back the weight and calories, hold your horses. Do it too fast or the wrong way, and you can get a serious and potentially life-threatening condition that occurs when a person who has been in a prolonged state of starvation or severe malnutrition begins to eat again. This condition results from the sudden shift in fluids and electrolytes that occurs when food intake is restarted after a period of nutritional deprivation. The metabolic changes that occur during refeeding can overwhelm the body, leading to dangerous complications, including heart failure, respiratory issues, and even death if not managed properly.

What Causes Refeeding Syndrome?

During prolonged starvation, the body adapts by slowing down metabolism and conserving resources. The body's main energy source shifts from glucose (sugar) to fat and muscle, leading to the breakdown of fat and protein stores for energy. This results in low levels of electrolytes such as **phosphate, magnesium, and potassium**, which are vital for many cellular functions.

When refeeding begins, especially with carbohydrates, insulin production spikes to help process the glucose from food. Insulin shifts electrolytes like phosphate, potassium, and magnesium from the blood into cells to facilitate cellular processes, which can lead to dangerously low levels of these electrolytes in the blood.

Key Risks in Refeeding Syndrome:

1. **Hypophosphatemia**: Low **phosphate** levels, which are critical for energy production in cells.
2. **Hypokalemia**: Low **potassium** levels, affecting heart and muscle function.
3. **Hypomagnesemia**: Low **magnesium** levels, impacting muscle and nerve function.
4. **Fluid Overload**: A shift in fluids can lead to heart failure or respiratory distress.
5. **Vitamin Deficiencies**: **Thiamine** (vitamin **B1**) is particularly crucial and is often deficient in malnourished individuals. Low thiamine can result in neurological problems (Wernicke's encephalopathy).

Symptoms of Refeeding Syndrome

- Fatigue
- Weakness
- Confusion
- Difficulty breathing
- High blood pressure
- Heart arrhythmias
- Seizures
- Coma (in severe cases)

How to Treat Refeeding Syndrome

1. **Slow and Controlled Refeeding**
   - Reintroduce calories gradually, starting with a low-calorie intake and increasing it slowly over several days or weeks. Initial intake should typically be 10-20 kcal/kg per day in high-risk individuals.
2. **Monitor Electrolytes**
   - Closely monitor serum phosphate, potassium, magnesium, and calcium levels daily, particularly during the first week of refeeding. Supplement these electrolytes as necessary.
3. **Thiamine Supplementation**
   - **Thiamine** (vitamin **B1**) should be supplemented before and during the refeeding process to prevent complications. Standard recommendations are 100-300 mg of thiamine daily before initiating refeeding, followed by ongoing supplementation.
4. **Fluid Management**
   - Careful fluid management is essential to prevent fluid overload. Fluids should be administered cautiously, and patients should be monitored for signs of fluid retention and heart failure.
5. **Multivitamin and Mineral Supplementation**
   - Along with thiamine, other vitamins (like B-complex and folate) and minerals should be supplemented to correct deficiencies and support metabolic recovery.
6. **Nutritional Support Team**
   - A team of healthcare providers, including **dietitians**, **nutritionists**, and **physicians** who are experts in this, should manage the refeeding process. Continuous monitoring and adjusting the refeeding plan based on the patient's response is crucial.

7. **Prevention**

   - **Risk Assessment**: Identify patients at high risk for refeeding syndrome, such as those who have experienced prolonged malnutrition, anorexia, chronic alcoholism, or post-surgery.
   - **Start Low, Go Slow**: Begin refeeding with caution, starting with lower calorie intakes and carefully monitoring vital signs and lab results.
   - **Electrolyte Daily Monitoring**
     - phosphate
     - potassium
     - magnesium

Gut Dysbiosis

Immune System Modulation

The gut microbiome is critical in modulating the immune system. However, Dysbiosis can disrupt this balance, leading to an overactive immune response and chronic inflammation. In Long COVID, gut dysbiosis may partially drive persistent immune activation and cytokine production.

Barrier Function

The integrity of the gut barrier is vital for preventing harmful substances from entering the bloodstream. Dysbiosis can compromise this barrier, leading to increased intestinal permeability, commonly known as "leaky gut." It allows bacterial endotoxins and other pro-inflammatory molecules to circulate systemically, potentially contributing to the prolonged inflammatory state observed in Long COVID.

Microbial Metabolites

The gut microbiome produces various metabolites, such as *Short-Chain Fatty Acids* (SCFAs), which have anti-inflammatory characteristics and support gut health. Dysbiosis can alter the production of these beneficial metabolites, further contributing to inflammation and disease.

Treating Gut Dysbiosis in Long COVID

1. **Prebiotics:** Prebiotics are non-digestible food ingredients that promote the growth of beneficial microorganisms in the intestines.
    - **Inulin**: Found in chicory root, garlic, and onions.
    - **Fructooligosaccharides (FOS)**: Present in fruits like bananas and vegetables such as asparagus.
    - **Galactooligosaccharides (GOS)**: It is found in dairy products and beans.
2. **Probiotics:** live microorganisms that, when administered in adequate amounts, confer a health benefit on the host
3. **Postbiotics:** Postbiotics are non-living bacterial products or metabolic byproducts from probiotics that exert biological activity in the host.
    - **Short-chain fatty acids (SCFAs)** include acetate, propionate, and butyrate.
    - **Enzymes**: These are produced during fermentation processes.
    - **Cell wall fragments**: From dead probiotic bacteria.
    - **Vitamins and peptides**: They are synthesized by probiotics.

Other Treatments:

- Apigenin
- BPC-157 (peptide)
- KPV-500 (peptide)
- Larazotide
- Butyrate

References:

- Zhang D, Zhou Y, Ma Y, Chen P, Tang J, Yang B, Li H, Liang M, Xue Y, Liu Y, Zhang J, Wang X. Gut Microbiota Dysbiosis Correlates with Long COVID-19 at One-Year After Discharge. J Korean Med Sci. 2023 Apr 17;38(15):e120. doi: 10.3346/jkms.2023.38.e120. PMID: 37069814; PMCID: PMC10111044.

- Clerbaux L-A, Filipovska J, Muñoz A, Petrillo M, Coecke S, Amorim M-J, Grenga L. Mechanisms Leading to Gut Dysbiosis in COVID-19: Current Evidence and Uncertainties Based on Adverse Outcome Pathways. *Journal of Clinical Medicine*. 2022; 11(18):5400. https://doi.org/10.3390/jcm11185400

- Giannos, P., & Prokopidis, K. (2022). Gut dysbiosis and long COVID-19: Feeling gutted. *Journal of Medical Virology*, 94. https://doi.org/10.1002/jmv.27684

Small Intestinal Bacterial Overgrowth – SIBO

Many gut microbiome resides in the colon. However, some also reside in the jejunum and ileum of the small intestine. When the population of the bacteria in the upper small intestine, called the duodenum, exceeds 10^5 organisms/ml, it can interfere with absorption, may acidify bile, or produce gas from carbohydrates and short-chain fatty acids. Some gram-negative coliforms, such as klebsiella, can damage the mucosa. It must be clear that our small intestines are not sterile. Are there any bacteria from the microbiome living there? However, due to the stomach's acidic environment, the small intestine's first part doesn't have high populations.

SIBO Symptoms

- Nausea
- Diarrhea
- Abdominal pain

Testing for Small Intestinal Bacterial Overgrowth (SIBO)

Breath Tests

- The most common and non-invasive way to diagnose SIBO. It involves consuming a sugar solution, usually **lactulose** or **glucose**, and then measuring the levels of **hydrogen** and **methane** gases in your breath over a period of time. Increased levels of these gases indicate bacterial overgrowth because bacteria in the small intestine ferment the sugar, producing these gases.

Small Intestine Aspirate and Culture

- This is a more invasive procedure that involves taking a fluid sample from the small intestine during an endoscopy. The fluid is then cultured to detect the presence of excessive bacteria. While considered the most accurate, it's less commonly used due to its invasive nature.

Other Diagnostic Methods

- **Blood tests** and **stool tests** may be used indirectly to assess nutrient deficiencies or fat malabsorption associated with SIBO, but they do not diagnose it directly.

The **lactulose breath test** is the most widely used due to its simplicity, but there can be limitations in its accuracy. If you're suspected of having SIBO, it's essential to work with a healthcare professional who can interpret the results alongside your symptoms.

What probiotics are safe to use with SIBO?

1. *Saccharomyces boulardii*

Safe Soil-Based Bacteria

- *Bacillus coagulans*
- *Bacillus subtilis* CU1 was generally safe and non-toxic in a clinical trial.
- *Bacillus clausii* (UBBC07) was generally safe and non-toxic for human use in a clinical trial.

Specific Probiotics

1. **Lactobacillus** and **Bifidobacterium** species are commonly used probiotics with proven efficacy in improving gut health and reducing inflammation.

2. ***Saccharomyces boulardii*** has shown promise in treating diarrhea and may benefit Long COVID patients with GI symptoms.

Prebiotics

Prebiotics are non-digestible food components that promote the growth and activity of beneficial gut bacteria. Common prebiotics include inulin, *fructooligosaccharides* (FOS), and *galactooligosaccharides* (GOS).

Dietary Sources

- Inulin is found in foods such as chicory root, garlic, onions, and bananas.

- FOS and GOS can be obtained from legumes, whole grains, and certain vegetables.

Diet plays a critical role in shaping the gut microbiome. A fiber-rich diet, polyphenols, and fermented foods can support a healthy microbiota and mitigate dysbiosis.

Specific Dietary Recommendations

- **Fiber:** Aim for a high-fiber diet with plenty of fruits, vegetables, legumes, and whole grains.

- **Polyphenols:** Include polyphenol-rich foods such as berries, green tea, dark chocolate, and red wine (in moderation).

- **Fermented Foods**: Incorporate fermented foods like yogurt, kefir (I suggest 8oz 2x/day), sauerkraut, kimchi, and miso, which provide beneficial probiotics.

Fecal Microbiota Transplantation (FMT)

FMT involves transferring stool from a healthy donor to a patient's gut with dysbiosis. This procedure can restore microbial diversity and has shown great promise in treating recurrent *Clostridioides difficile (C. diff)* infections and other GI disorders. Ongoing research studies are striving to evaluate its efficacy in Long COVID.

In addition to dietary changes, lifestyle modifications can support gut health and reduce dysbiosis.

- **Stress Management:** Chronic stress can adversely impact the gut microbiome. However, techniques such as mindfulness, meditation, yoga, and regular physical activity can help manage stress.

- **Sleep Hygiene:** Poor sleep can disrupt the gut microbiome. Aim for 7-9 hours of quality sleep per night and maintain a regular sleep schedule.

- **Avoiding Unnecessary Antibiotics:** Antibiotics can significantly disrupt the gut microbiota. You can use them only when necessary and under the guidance of a healthcare professional. Disclaimer: If you are fighting a bacterial infection elsewhere, the need for this outweighs the risk to the microbiome.

Other Treatments

An antibiotic such as **rifaximin** may be needed to reduce the microbiome population in the small intestine.

References:

- Achufusi TGO, Sharma A, Zamora EA, Manocha D. Small Intestinal Bacterial Overgrowth: Comprehensive Review of Diagnosis, Prevention, and Treatment Methods. Cureus. 2020 Jun 27;12(6):e8860. doi: 10.7759/cureus.8860. PMID: 32754400; PMCID: PMC7386065.

- Rao, Satish S. C. MD, PhD; Bhagatwala, Jigar MBBS, MPH[1]. Small Intestinal Bacterial Overgrowth: Clinical Features and Therapeutic Management. Clinical and Translational Gastroenterology 10(10):p e00078, October 2019. | DOI: 10.14309/ctg.0000000000000078

- Pimentel, Mark MD, FRCP(C), FACG; Saad, Richard J. MD, FACG; Long, Millie D. MD, MPH, FACG (GRADE Methodologist); Rao, Satish S. C. MD, PhD, FRCP, FACG. ACG Clinical Guideline: Small Intestinal Bacterial Overgrowth. The American Journal of Gastroenterology 115(2):p 165-178, February 2020. | DOI: 10.14309/ajg.0000000000000501

- Rezaie, A., Buresi, M., Lembo, A., et al. (2017). Hydrogen and Methane-Based Breath Testing in Gastrointestinal Disorders: The North American Consensus. *The American Journal of Gastroenterology, 112*(5), 775–784. https://doi.org/10.1038/ajg.2017.46

Ehlers-Danlos Syndrome (EDS)

Ehlers-Danlos Syndrome (EDS) is a group of genetic disorders that influence connective tissues, which provide strength and elasticity to structures like skin, joints, and blood vessels. This condition is not typical, but it is mentioned here because you can acquire several EDS attributes from Long COVID. This situation may be due to the elastase enzyme released from mast cells, which softens tissues. It is also a risk factor for Long COVID because it can cause dysautonomia. Long COVID does NOT cause EDS but can result in a hypermobility-like effect. In my opinion, it is from mast cell release of an enzyme called **elastase**. Elastase is an enzyme that breaks down elastin, a protein that makes tissues stretchy. When there is **less elastase**, your skin can't spring back after stretching. It makes skin saggier.

Key Features of EDS

- **Hypermobile Joints:** People with EDS often have flexible joints that move beyond the normal range. It can lead to frequent dislocations and joint pain.
- **Skin Elasticity:** Their skin may easily be unusually stretchy, fragile, and bruised.
- **Chronic Pain:** Many individuals experience ongoing pain in their muscles and joints.
- **Poor Wound Healing:** They might have problems with wound healing and scar formation.
- **Dysautonomia**

- **Craniocervical instability (CCI)** is a medical condition where the strong ligaments that hold your head to your upper neck are loose or lax.
  - **Head and Neck Pain**: Patients often describe a sensation of heaviness in the head, sometimes feeling like a "*bobblehead*."
  - **Balance Issues**: Problems with coordination and maintaining balance.
  - **Dizziness and Vertigo**: Experiencing spinning sensations or lightheadedness.
  - **Vision Problems**: Blurred vision, reduced visual acuity, or changes in peripheral vision.
  - **Neurological Symptoms**: Issues with swallowing or speaking, among other neurological issues.
  - **Other Symptoms:** include headaches, muscle weakness, nausea, vomiting, irregular eye movements, or persistent fatigue.
  - **Treatment:** these ligaments can be tightened with regenerative therapy and prolotherapy.

References:

- Miklovic T, Sieg VC. Ehlers-Danlos Syndrome. [Updated 2023 May 29]. In: StatPearls [Internet]. Treasure Island (FL): StatPearls Publishing; 2024 Jan-. Available from: https://www.ncbi.nlm.nih.gov/books/NBK549814/

- Schubart JR, Mills SE, Francomano CA, Stuckey-Peyrot H. A qualitative study of pain and related symptoms experienced by people with Ehlers-Danlos syndromes. Front Med (Lausanne). 2024 Jan 3;10:1291189. doi: 10.3389/fmed.2023.1291189. PMID: 38235272; PMCID: PMC10792024.

- Lohkamp LN, Marathe N, Fehlings MG. Craniocervical Instability in Ehlers-Danlos Syndrome-A Systematic Review of Diagnostic and Surgical Treatment Criteria. Global Spine J. 2022 Oct;12(8):1862-1871. doi: 10.1177/21925682211068520. Epub 2022 Feb 23. PMID: 35195459; PMCID: PMC9609512.

REACTIVATION of Infections

While I do not believe that these infections cause Long COVID, Long COVID can cause a relapse or reactivation. These reactivations need to be treated separately outside of Long COVID.

Epstein-Barr Virus (EBV) Reactivation

Epstein-Barr Virus (EBV) is the virus that causes infectious mononucleosis (mono) and can reactivate in some individuals, especially those with weakened immune systems.

Symptoms of EBV reactivation

- **Fatigue**: Profound, often debilitating tiredness.
- **Fever**: Low-grade fever.
- **Sore Throat**: Persistent sore throat, sometimes with swollen tonsils.
- **Swollen Lymph Nodes**: Particularly in the neck.
- **Headaches**: Persistent and severe headaches.
- **Muscle Aches**: Generalized muscle pain.
- **Night Sweats**: Episodes of excessive sweating during sleep.
- **Rash**: In some cases, a rash can develop.
- **Liver Dysfunction**: Mild liver enzyme elevations.
- **Spleen Enlargement**: Sometimes, the spleen can be enlarged.

Laboratory Tests

	VCA IgM	VCA IgG = for life	EA = active	EBNA = for life
Susceptible to infection	-	-	-	-
Early and primary infection	+	+	-	-
Active infection	+ or -	+	+	-
Past infection	-	+	-	+
Reactivation	+ or -	+	+	+

A. Bloodwork (Antibody Testing)

Antibodies to various parts of the EBV virus are used to determine the stage of EBV infection (acute, past, or reactivation) by detecting different types of antibodies produced against the virus:

- **EBV Viral Capsid Antigen (VCA) IgM and IgG, antibodies**
    - **IgM**: Typically indicates recent infection, present in the early stages.
    - **IgG**: Indicates past infection or long-term immunity.
- **EBV Nuclear Antigen (EBNA) IgG antibody**
    - Appears later during the infection (2-4 months after the initial infection) and persists for life.

  - Its presence without VCA IgM suggests past infection or reactivation.

- **Early Antigen (EA) IgG, antibody**
  - **Positive EA IgG** suggests active or reactivated EBV.
  - This marker is often elevated in EBV reactivation.
  - Falls after 3-6 months after infection to undetectable.

B. EBV DNA Quantification (PCR)

- **Polymerase Chain Reaction (PCR)** can measure EBV DNA levels in the blood or tissues.
- **High viral loads** detected by PCR are indicative of reactivation, especially in immunocompromised individuals or in severe cases of reactivation.
- PCR is particularly useful for identifying EBV in various tissues (e.g., liver, lungs, brain) or bodily fluids like cerebrospinal fluid (CSF), depending on symptoms.

C. Complete Blood Count (CBC) and Liver Function Tests

- **Atypical lymphocytes** or **lymphocytosis** (an increase in lymphocytes) are common findings in active EBV infection.
- Elevated **liver enzymes** (e.g., ALT, AST) can indicate liver involvement, which is frequent in both acute infection and reactivation.

E. Heterophile Antibody Test (Monospot)

- Commonly used for diagnosing **acute** mononucleosis but less useful for detecting reactivation (don't use to see if you have EBV reactivation).

Most reactivations are asymptomatic. Long COVID is associated with EBV reactivation.

Treatment is targeted against active EBV replication if the symptoms are troublesome or rare complications transpire, such as encephalomyelitis, cerebellar ataxia, lymphoma, or multiple *sclerosis*. No EBV treatments have been approved on-label by the FDA. **Off-label**, several options exist:

- **acyclovir** – Zovirax
- **ganciclovir** – Zirgan
- **valacyclovir** - Valtrex
- **valganciclovir** – Valcyte
- **Cidofovir** - Vistide
- **Dipyridamole** – this one can also prevent reactivations, by suppressing nucleoside uptake and suppressing EBV gene expression.

References:

- Thomé MP, Borde C, Larsen AK, Henriques JAP, Lenz G, Escargueil AE, Maréchal V. Dipyridamole as a new drug to prevent Epstein-Barr virus reactivation. Antiviral Res. 2019 Dec;172:104615. DOI: 10.1016/j.antiviral.2019.104615. Epub 2019 Sep 30. PMID: 31580916.
- Andrei G, Trompet E, Snoeck R. Novel Therapeutics for Epstein-Barr Virus. Molecules. 2019 Mar 12;24(5):997. DOI: 10.3390/molecules24050997. PMID: 30871092; PMCID: PMC6429425.
- Bernal KDE, Whitehurst CB. Incidence of Epstein-Barr virus reactivation is elevated in COVID-19 patients. Virus Res. 2023 Sep;334:199157. doi: 10.1016/j.virusres.2023.199157. Epub 2023 Jun 26. PMID: 37364815; PMCID: PMC10292739.
- Hoeggerl, A.D., Nunhofer, V., Lauth, W. *et al.* Epstein-Barr virus reactivation is not causative for post-COVID-19-syndrome in individuals with asymptomatic or mild SARS-CoV-2 disease course. *BMC Infect Dis* **23**, 800 (2023). https://doi.org/10.1186/s12879-023-08820-w
- Peluso, M. J., Deveau, T.-M., Munter, S. E., Ryder, D., Buck, A., Beck-Engeser, G., Chan, F., Lu, S., Goldberg, S. A., Hoh, R., Tai, V., Torres, L., Iyer, N. S., Deswal, M., Ngo, L. H., Buitrago, M., Rodriguez, A., Chen, J. Y., Yee, B. C., ... Henrich, T. J. (2023). Impact of pre-existing chronic viral infection and reactivation on the development of Long COVID. *Journal of Clinical Investigation*, 133(15), e163669. https://doi.org/10.1172/JCI163669

- Thomé, M. P., Borde, C., Larsen, A. K., Henriques, J. A. P., Lenz, G., Escargueil, A. E., & Maréchal, V. (2019). Dipyridamole as a new drug to prevent Epstein-Barr virus reactivation. *Antiviral Research, 172,* 104615. https://doi.org/10.1016/j.antiviral.2019.104615

Lyme Disease

Lyme disease is caused by the bacterium *Borrelia burgdorferi* and is typically transmitted by tick bites. Symptoms of this disease can vary depending on the stage of infection:

1. **Early Localized Stage** (days to weeks after tick bite):
    - **Erythema Migrans**: It is also called *Bull's-Eye* Rash. It is typically a red rash that expands over several days, sometimes clearing in the center.
    - **Flu-Like Symptoms**: Fever, chills, headache, fatigue, muscle and joint aches, swollen lymph nodes.
2. **Early Disseminated Stage** (weeks to months after tick bite):
    - **Additional Rashes**: Similar to erythema migrans, but not at the bite site.
    - **Neurological Symptoms**: It can cause facial palsy (loss of muscle tone or droop on one or both sides of the face) and meningitis-like symptoms, including severe headaches and neck stiffness.
    - **Cardiac Symptoms** include heart palpitations and irregular heartbeat (Lyme carditis).
3. **Late Disseminated Stage** (months to years after tick bite):
    - **Arthritis**: Severe joint pain and swelling, especially in the knees.
    - **Neurological Issues** include neuropathy, memory problems, and cognitive challenges.
4. **Post-Treatment Lyme Disease Syndrome (PTLDS)** describes *Lyme* disease patients who have the infection cleared by antibiotics but then experience persisting symptoms of pain, fatigue, or cognitive impairment. Currently, little is known about the cause or epidemiology of PTLDS.

References:

- Chung, M. K., Caboni, M., Strandwitz, P., D'Onofrio, A., Lewis, K., & Patel, C. J. (2023). Systematic comparisons between Lyme disease and post-treatment Lyme disease syndrome in the U.S. with administrative claims data. *EBioMedicine*, 89, 104524. https://DOI.org/10.1016/j.ebiom.2023.104524

Pediatric Long COVID

Symptoms in Children

Long COVID can influence children differently than adults, with symptoms such as fatigue, headaches, and abdominal pain. Young children may have a challenging time verbalizing that they feel sick. Even though Long COVID is less common in children compared to adults, studies show that approximately 10-20% of children who were infected with COVID will develop symptoms within 6 months of recovery. Similar to how adults with Long COVID get treated, children can be mocked by their friends, school nurses, and teachers who are told over and over to their faces that there is nothing wrong with them and to stop faking it. Keep in mind that especially younger children will not be able to express what they are feeling and it makes diagnosis Long COVID that much more difficult.

Diagnostic Challenges

Diagnosing Long COVID in children has unique challenges, including the overlap with other pediatric conditions. This section evaluates diagnostic tools and techniques for pediatric patients.

Symptoms

1. **Fatigue**: Persistent tiredness that doesn't improve with rest and affects daily activities.
2. **Respiratory Issues**: Shortness of breath, cough, and chest pain are common respiratory complaints.

3. **Neurological Symptoms** include headaches, difficulty concentrating (often called "brain fog"), dizziness, and sleep disturbances.
4. **Gastrointestinal Problems** include abdominal pain, nausea, diarrhea, and loss of appetite.
5. **Musculoskeletal Pain**: Joint and muscle pain.
6. **Mental Health Issues** include anxiety, depression, and mood swings.
7. **Cardiovascular Symptoms** involve palpitations and chest pain.
8. **Multisystem Inflammatory Syndrome in Children (MIS-C)**: It is a severe but less common condition occurring after COVID-19 infection and is characterized by inflammation affecting multiple organ systems.

Symptoms to monitor in young children

- Trouble with memory or focusing
- Back or neck pain
- Stomach pain
- Headache
- Phobias
- Refusing to go to school
- Itchy skin or rash
- Trouble sleeping
- Nausea or vomiting
- Feeling lightheaded or dizzy

In adolescents, monitor for these symptoms

- Change in or loss of smell and/or taste
- Body, muscle or joint pain
- Daytime tiredness

- Fatigue after walking
- Back or neck pain
- Trouble with memory or focusing
- Headache
- Feeling lightheaded or dizzy

Diagnosis

- **Clinical Evaluation**: Comprehensive medical history and physical examination.
- **Laboratory Tests**: Blood tests to rule out other causes of symptoms.
- **Imaging Studies**: Chest X-rays or CT scans if respiratory symptoms are present.
- **Specialist Referral**: Consulting pediatricians, neurologists, cardiologists, or other specialists as required.

Management

- **Multidisciplinary Approach**: It involves various healthcare professionals such as pediatricians, physiotherapists, psychologists, and dietitians.
- **Symptomatic Treatment**: The treatment process incorporates medications for pain, breathing exercises for respiratory issues, and counseling for mental health support.
- **Rehabilitation**: Physical therapy to help with fatigue and muscle weakness.
- **Nutritional Support**: Ensuring a balanced diet to support overall health and recovery.
- **School Support**: Adjustments in school to accommodate the child's tailored needs, such as modified schedules or supplementary academic support.

Prognosis

The prognosis for children with Long COVID varies. While many children gradually improve, some may experience persistent symptoms for months. Ongoing research is crucial to better understand the long-term impact and to develop tailored and patient-oriented treatments.

References:

1. Harris E. Millions of US Children Experience Range of Long COVID Effects. *JAMA.* 2024;331(9):726.

   DOI:10.1001/jama.2024.0356

2. Gross RS, Thaweethai T, Kleinman LC, et al. Characterizing Long COVID in Children and Adolescents. *JAMA.* Published online August 21, 2024. DOI:10.1001/jama.2024.12747

Putting It All Together

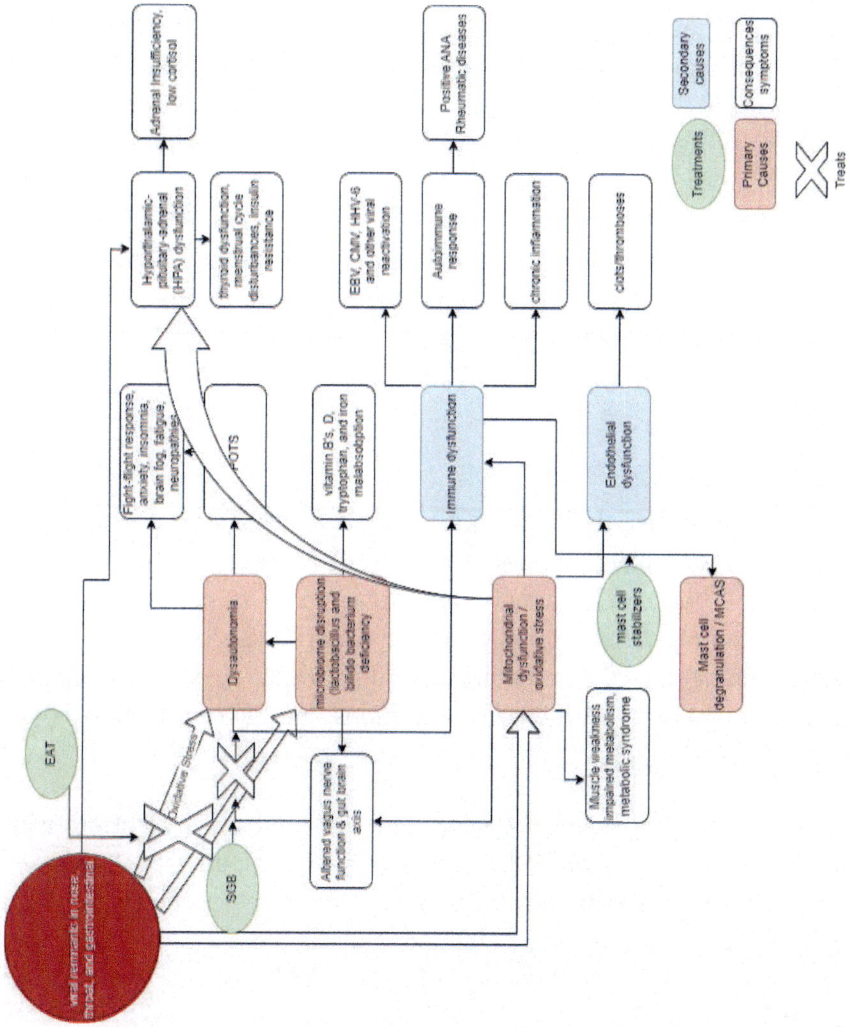

Conclusion

Long COVID has manifested itself as a stain on most of the world, with more than 17 million *Americans* and 57 million worldwide suffering from it. I suspect there are 10 times more who have not come forward. As we conclude this comprehensive journey through understanding Long COVID, we must reflect on the resilience, determination, and hope that signifies the human spirit. Patients suffering from Long COVID have endured unprecedented challenges. The pandemic influenced countless lives with persistent symptoms that often seem insurmountable. However, through the collective efforts of patients, healthcare practitioners, researchers, and advocates, we have made significant strides toward understanding and managing this intricate condition.

The successes shared in this book signify the struggles and triumphs of individuals who have endured Long COVID head-on. Their experiences underscore the importance of a holistic approach to health, considering recovery's physical, emotional, and psychological aspects. It is evident that overcoming Long COVID requires a multidisciplinary effort, integrating medical treatments with lifestyle variations, mental health support, and community resources.

Research rapidly evolves, bringing new and in-depth insights into the mechanisms behind Long COVID and potential therapeutic approaches. As our knowledge expands, so does our ability to provide effective treatments and support for those affected. Consequently, the promising advancements in medical science offer hope for better management and, eventually, a cure.

For patients, persistence and self-advocacy remain critical. It is essential to stay informed, seek out supportive healthcare professionals, and connect with others encountering similar challenges. Building a solid support network can provide emotional strength and practical advice, making the journey toward recovery less daunting.

Healthcare practitioners play a vital role in this journey. Empathy, active listening, avoiding gaslighting, and a patient-centered approach are imperative in addressing the unique needs of Long COVID patients. Continued education and collaboration among medical professionals will ensure that patients receive the best care possible.

For researchers, the quest for answers continues—the complexities of Long COVID demand innovative research techniques and interdisciplinary collaboration. Persistent funding and support for Long COVID research are imperative to unraveling the mysteries of this condition and developing effective treatments.

As a society, we must recognize the impact of Long COVID and provide the necessary resources to support the affected individuals. For instance, public awareness, policy changes, and funding for research studies and healthcare services are critical components in addressing the long-term implications of this pandemic.

In conclusion, while the road to recovery from Long COVID might be protracted and challenging, it is navigable, manageable, and, most importantly, treatable. With perseverance, empathy, and a combined effort, we can overcome the impediments of Long COVID and emerge stronger. This journey is a testament to the strength of the human spirit and the power of collective action. Together, we can pave the way for a future where Long COVID is no longer a daunting specter but a manageable chapter in human health's long and winding story.

Printed in Great Britain
by Amazon

56726878R00185